Study Guide

Animal Care

Level 2 Technical - Exam 024/524

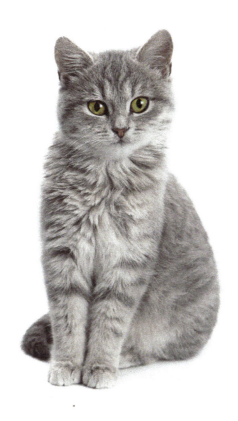

The publisher gratefully acknowledges the permission of copyright holders to reproduce copyright material:

p7 ©Alexandr Ermolaev©123RF.com; p.12 (left) dimarik16©123RF.com; (right) andriano©123RF.com; p.13 (left) Thanayu Jongwattanasilkul©123RF.com; (right) iStock.com/Henrik_L; p.30 (top left) PENCHAN PUMILA©123RF.com; (bottom left) areeya©123RF.com ; (bottom right) mtsaride©123RF.com; p.39 vladdon©123RF.com; p.43 (left) Dmitry Kalinovsky©123RF.com; (right) Alexander Kharchenko©123RF.com; p.44 Anja Seibert©123RF.com; p.50 pryzmat©123RF.com; p.56 millions27©123RF.com; p.61 Dirk Ercken©123RF.com; p.62 imagemax©123RF.com; p.66 (left) Santiago Nunez Iniguez©123RF.com; (right) serezniy©123RF.com; p.68 Anton Starikov©123RF.com; p.72 kzenon ©123RF.com; p.88 M Schaefer©123RF.com; p.97 Ruud Morijn©123RF.com; p.100 okssi68©123RF.com; p.102 jessinono©123RF.com; p.109 Anton Gvozdikov©123RF.com; p.117 Olga Volodina©123RF.com

Cover image: Leonid Nyshko©123RF.com

All other photographs and illustrations are © Eboru Publishing.

Every effort has been made to trace copyright holders and to obtain their permission for the use of copyright material. The publisher will be glad to make arrangements with any copyright holder it has not been possible to contact.

Copyright © 2020 Eboru Publishing

First edition 2020.

ISBN 978-0-9929002-4-3

Ordering Information

Special discounts are available for class set purchases by schools, colleges and others. For details, contact the publisher at: enquiries@eboru.com

Trade orders: copies of this book are available through the normal wholesalers.

For any queries please contact: orders@eboru.com

www.eboru.com

Features in this book

Topic introduction
Brief summary of what you will cover in the next section.

In this topic you will learn about:

- Frequency of monitoring signs of health.

- Frequency of the following regimes: feeding, water exercise, grooming.

- Cleaning of accommodation including fixtures and fittings, partial and total clean.

Quiz Questions
Knowledge-check questions at the end of each section, so that you can quickly recap on what you have learned.

Quiz Questions

1 a) How might the appearance of an animal's coat be a sign of ill health?
   b) What might be a behavioural sign of poor health?

2 What does the term respiration mean?

Jargon Buster
There are lots of technical and specialist terms that you will come across whilst studying. This feature will explain what these specialist words mean.

Jargon Buster
gait the movement of the limbs as the animal walks or runs

Activity
Tasks that will help you build your knowledge and understanding of the subject.

Activity

Research some common vocalisations in two animals of your choice.

Book Order Details	
Order No:	934768
Date:	July 2022
Supplier:	Browns
Cost:	£16·99
Barcode No:	R70423
Class No:	636·089

3

Contents

Answers to questions are available by subscribing to our email updates at www.eboru.com

Unit 201 Maintain animal health and welfare

LO1 Monitor and maintain the health of animals

1.1 Signs of health in animals, incorporating routine health checks

In this topic you will learn about:

- **Signs of health: behaviour; movement and gait; appearance of eyes, ears, nose, mouth, teeth, mucous membranes; Appearance of coat, limbs, feet, faeces, urine; weight / condition; food and water intake.**

- **Normal parameters for temperature, pulse and respiration.**

- **Frequency of monitoring signs of health.**

- **Frequency of the following regimes: feeding, water exercise, grooming.**

- **Cleaning of accommodation including fixtures and fittings, partial and total clean.**

- **Recording methods.**

Signs of health

Behaviour

Each species of animal has different behavioural traits and individual animals within a species might also behave slightly differently. Behaviour that is unusal for that species or unusual for that animal can indicate health problems. You can ask yourself the following questions:

- Is there a change in the animal's temperament?

- Are they quieter, more timid or more fearful than normal?

- Are they more aggressive than normal?

- Do they appear to be in any pain?

Movement and gait

Awkward or restrictive movements might indicate an injury:

- Is the animal moving normally?

- Do they appear to have any restrictive movements?

- Does their posture look normal?

- Does their gait look normal – are their limbs co-ordinated, are they staggering, shuffling or missing a stride?

Appearance of eyes, ears, nose, mouth/teeth, mucous membranes

- Are the eyes bright, clear and free from cloudiness?

- Are the ears free of any unusual

discharge?

- Is the nose free of any unusual discharge? Is the nose in good condition?
- Are the mouth and teeth in good condition? Are they a normal colour? Are there any unusual smells?

The gums or the tongue are good places to assess the condition of the mucous membrane. The following colours can indicate the following:

- A white mucous membrane may mean the animal is in shock, or has a low count of red blood cells due to bleeding.
- A pink mucous membrane is normal.
- A red mucous membrane can be a sign of an infection or heat stroke.
- A blue mucous membrane is a sign of low oxygen content in the blood.
- A yellow mucous membrane is a sign that there may be a liver or kidney problem.

Appearance of coat, limbs/feet, faeces, urine

- Is the fur or coat glossy and healthy in appearance?
- Is the fur matted or in bad condition?
- Are there any visible sores, broken skin or other damage?
- Is there any evidence of lick marks (which is a sign of good health)?

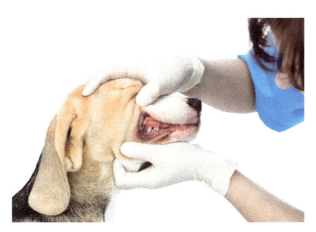

Figure 1 Examining a dog's gums

- Is the animal walking freely or limping?
- Is the animal using all limbs equally?
- Are there any areas of swelling?
- Are the feet or hooves in good condition, without sores or signs of infection?
- Are the claws in good condition, not overly long or twisted out of shape?

- What colour is the urine?
- Is there a change in the consistency of faeces?
- Is the animal passing faeces or urine more or less often than normal?

Weight/condition

- Is the animal over or underweight?
- Is the animal rapidly gaining or losing weight?

Food and water intake

Changes to an animal's appetite can indicate a number of different health conditions.

- Has the animal eaten a normal amount of food and water since the last time they were fed?
- Has the animal's appetite changed?

Normal parameters for temperature, pulse and respiration

Temperature

It is generally accepted that rectal thermometers provide the most accurate readings. You can use digital thermometers or mercury thermometers. A digital thermometer will make a sound once an accurate temperature has been measured and displays the temperature as a number. When using a mercury thermometer you need to wait for the mercury to stop moving and then read the temperature from the scale.

To take a temperature reading:

- add lubricant to the measurement probe

- lift the animal's tail and insert the probe into the rectum

- wait until you hear a beep (digital) or until the reading has stabilised (mercury) then read the and record the measurement

- remove the probe, clean and disinfect.

As you will be assisting someone make sure to follow all of their instructions.

Normal Rectal Temperature Ranges	Temperature in Celcius
Cow	36.7–39.3
Cat	38.1–39.2
Dog	37.9–39.9
Horse	37.2 - 38.3
Pig	38.7–39.8
Rabbit	38.6–40.1
Hamster	36.1–38.9

Adapted from Robertshaw D. Temperature Regulation and Thermal Environment, in Dukes' Physiology of Domestic Animals, 12th ed., Reece WO, Ed. Copyright 2004 by Cornell University.

Pulse rate

You can take a pulse by locating a major artery and lightly pressing your index and middle finger against it. The best location is different for each animal but some common locations are:

- horse: the jaw/cheek

- dog: at the top of inside back leg

- cat: at the top of inside back leg

- cattle: underneath the base of the tail

- pigs: at the top of inside back leg

- hamster: just behind the elbows, using a forefinger and thumb.

You can count the beats over a full minute, or count over 30 seconds and multiply by two.

Normal pulse rate values	Beats per minute
Cow	48–84
Cat	120–140
Dog	70–120
Horse	28–40
Pig	70–120
Rabbit	180–350
Hamster	300–600

Adapted from Detweiler DK and Erickson HH, Regulation of the Heart, in Dukes' Physiology of Domestic Animals, 12th ed., Reece WO, Ed. Copyright 2004 by Cornell University.

Respiration rate

You can measure respiration – i.e. breathing – by either counting the rise and fall of the animal's chest visually, or you can place your hand on the flank of the animal and count it that way. You need to count the number of breaths over a minute.

Typical respiration rates	Rate per minute
Cat	16–40
Dairy cow	26–50
Dog	18–34
Horse	10–14
Pig	32–58
Hamster	34–114

Adapted from Reece WO, Respiration in Mammals, in Dukes' Physiology of Domestic Animals, 12th ed., Reece WO, Ed. Copyright 2004 by Cornell University.

Frequency of monitoring signs of health

Daily checks

- Appetite and water intake.

- Faeces and urine.

- Behaviour.

- Movement and gait.

Weekly checks

- Eyes, ears, nose, mouth and teeth.
- Coat, fur and skin.
- Mucous membranes.
- Limbs and feet.
- Genitals and anal area.

Monthly checks

- General conditon of body.
- Weight check.

Frequency of the following regimes

The frequency of the following means how often they should be done.

Feeding

How often you should feed an animals is very dependent on species. However most mammals would normally be fed at least once per day.

Water

All animals need water to survive. A lack of water can quickly become life-threatening for most animals. So it is critical that fresh and clean drinking water is available for animals at all times.

For animals that partly or wholly live in water, it is essential that the water acidity and alkalinity is kept within an acceptable range. Most animals will need water that is neither acidic or alkali. There must be an adequate monitoring system in place to enure this.

Water in fish tanks should be changed every 1-2 weeks but this depends on how many fish are in the tank.

Exercise

Most animals require a certain amount of daily exercise. Most animals' wild ancestors or counterparts would normally spend a good deal of time moving in order to find food.

Different species and breeds require different amounts of exercise. Animals of the same species and breed but with different lifestyles would also require different amounts of planned exercise. For instance a working dog is unlikely to need a large amount of additional planned exercise.

It is important that you understand what is considered to be a normal amount of exercise for the species and lifestyle of the animal you are considering.

Grooming

Frequency of grooming is dependent on the coat and fur of the animal in question, and to some extent how well they can clean themselves. There are no hard and fast rules but in dogs, for instance, smooth and short-haired breeds need less regular grooming than thicker or silkier long-haired breeds. It would be normal for dogs such as spaniels and poodles to need grooming once a day.

Similarly, whilst cats are better at self-grooming than dogs, short-haired cats need less grooming (around twice per week) than long-haired cats, which might need grooming once per day.

> **Activity**
>
> What are typical feeding, exercise and grooming frequencies for your chosen species?

Cleaning of accommodation

It is important that an animal's living areas are kept clean and hygienic, to prevent disease and illness. They must also be free of hazards in order to keep the animal safe.

- **Disinfection:** animals can be a source of germs (also known as pathogens). This may be through contact with other animals as well as from faeces and urine left in their living areas. This is particularly true if there are different animals sharing the same space.

- **Fixtures and fittings:** equipment must be cleaned to ensure it is safe for animals to use. All equipment should be cleaned weekly but some will need to be cleaned much more often - for instance, water containers or bottles need a full clean each day.

- **Partial and total clean:** a partial clean should be undertaken every day or more often if required. On top of this a thorough 'total' clean should be done every week.

Recording methods

Conducting the health checks mentioned above is of little value unless findings are recorded. This allows you to monitor changes over time and also gives everyone access to an animal's current and previous health status.

Recordings may be paper-based, entered into a computer, or both. It is important for all relevant people to know where the records are and for everyone to record information using the same questions or prompts. Some checks are daily, some are weekly, some are monthly, and others may be even more or less frequent than this. Each observation should be recorded by everyone in line with these timings.

It is important that recordings of observations are accurate so that any likely health issues can be identified and addressed. Observations should also use consistent criteria, particularly as different people might observe the same animal. For instance, if a scale of 1 to 5 is used to describe how healthy an animal's coat looks, everyone needs to use the same scale and know that 5 means 'very healthy'.

Jargon Buster

frequency how often something happens

gait the movement of the limbs as an animal walks or runs

mucous membrane a layer of cells that surrounds certain organs and openings in the body. Such openings include the inner nose, mouth and tongue. The membrane often secretes a fluid, known as mucous. The mucous membrane protects those areas from infection and stops them from drying out.

pathogen very small organisms that cause disease

respiration breathing

Quiz Questions

1 a) How might the appearance of an animal's coat be a sign of ill health? b) What might be a behavioural sign of poor health?

2 What does the term respiration mean?

3 Why is cleaning important?

1.2 Routine preventative applications and treatments for animals

In this topic you will learn about:

- **Identification and treatment of internal and external parasites**

- **Routine care and procedures: foot care, mouth/dental care, ear care, species or breed-specific needs, grooming and skin/scale care, eyes, weighing.**

Parasites

A parasite is any organism that lives on or in another organism, which is called the host. Parasites get their food from their host. Internal parasites live in an animal, e.g. worms. and external parasites live on an animal, e.g. fleas, ticks, mites, lice.

Different species of animals attract particular parasites. There are different treatments available for different parasites and for different species but they can be split into the following:

- Topical: these are treatments applied to the surface of the body, such as the skin or eyes. These treatments include creams, lotions, shampoos and sprays.

- Oral: these are treatments that are given by mouth either in feed, water, or as tablets.

Worms

Worms are organisms that can live within an animal's body. There are two main types of worm:

- roundworms – these are round, white, and grow up to 15cm long

- tapeworms – these are flat, consisting of a head with a body made of independent segments, and grow up to 60cm long

Both of these normally live in the animal's small intestine.

Symptoms of worms are:

- presence of worms in faeces or vomit – roundworms look like small white pieces of string, whilst fragments of tapeworms look like or small grains of rice

- diarrhoea

- anaemia

- dehydration

- loss of weight

- pot belly

- behaviour indicating an itching anus.

However these may only appear when the infestation is advanced. Prior to that there may not be any obvious symptoms.

It is not uncommon for young puppies to already have roundworms and hence puppies and kittens need worming.

Some tapeworms can be passed on to humans so you must always thoroughly wash your hands and disinfect surfaces after treatment.

Treatment of worms: normally through de-worming medication – either tablets, injections or spots on the collar. Puppies and kittens need worming as it is quite common for them to become infected by their mothers when in the womb.

Prevention of worms: keep animals free from fleas, dispose of faeces promptly, restrict animals' movement outdoors in order to avoid areas with droppings.

Fleas

Fleas live on the skin and feed off the animal's blood.

Symptoms of fleas are:

- skin irritation

- other allergic reactions

- blood infections.

Evidence for fleas is flea 'dirt' – digested blood excreted by adult fleas, which can be seen by combing the animal's coat onto white paper and looking for dark red or brown specs.

Fleas can also carry other pathogenic organisms which cause more serious problems. For instance fleas carry the deadly rabbit disease myxomatosis.

Treatment of fleas: there are a few methods to treat fleas - sprays, powders, tablets and shampoos are all available to treat the animal. However a large percentage of the flea population consists of eggs and larvae. Therefore it is advisable to vacuum, clean and treat the environment as well.

Prevention of fleas: normally using tablets, collars, shampoos and sprays that contain ingredients that are toxic for fleas.

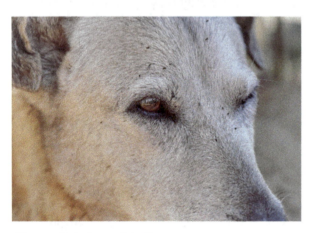

Figure 2 A dog with fleas

Ticks

Ticks move from one host to another and feed off each host's blood.

Symptoms of ticks are:

- itching and skin irritation
- loss of fur
- dull coat.

Ticks can carry diseases which they pass to the host, including Lyme disease, whose symptoms include lameness or seemingly arthritic joints.

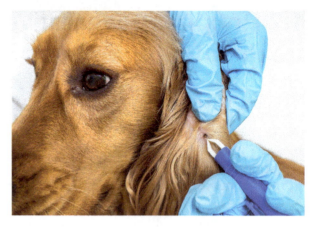

Figure 3 A dog tick being removed

Treatment of ticks: as with fleas, there are a range of sprays, powders, tablets, collars and shampoos available.

If a tick is found on an animal it can be removed using specialist equipment. However it is important that ticks are not pulled out as they can leave their mouths embedded in the animal and cause further infection.

Prevention of ticks: can be as simple as keeping an animal indoors or restricting their movement when outside. Higher-risk environments include wooded and vegetated areas.

Mites

Mites are similar to ticks but tend to be smaller. They either feed on organic material, like dead skin, or the host's blood. They either live on the surface of the skin or burrow just underneath. It is less common for mites to carry diseases.

Symptoms of mites are:

- itchiness
- sore, dry skin
- dark crusts of skin in the ears can indicate the presence of ear mites
- poor condition, due to the skin disease mange which is caused by mites.

Treatment of mites: chemicals that kill mites and ticks are available in sprays, dips, shampoos etc.

Prevention of mites: keeping bedding and the environment clean will help to prevent mites

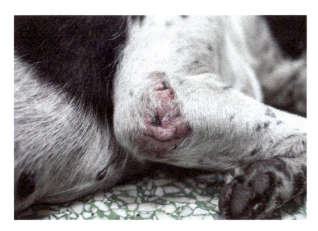

Figure 4 A dog with mange caused by mites

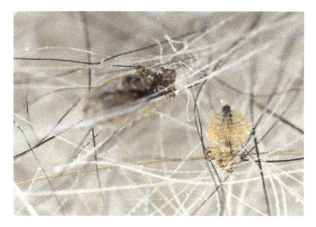

Figure 5 A closeup image of a dog with lice

but separating infected and non-infected animals is key.

Lice

Lice are under 5 mm long and are split into 'bloodsucking' and 'biting'. Lice can only live on one species, meaning that lice cannot spread from one species to another.

Symptoms of lice are:

- itching
- bad skin condition
- loss of hair or fur.

Treatment of lice: shampoos, powders and sprays are all available to treat the animal and its environment.

Prevention of lice: lice can only survive on the host, and rely on host-to-host contact to spread. So, preventing lice can be as simple as ensuring that animals are closely checked before coming into contact with clean animals, and equipment such as combs and bedding are not shared with infected or unchecked animals.

Routine care and procedures appropriate for species

Foot care

Dogs and cats

Check that the nails have not overgrown - are they dragging along the floor? Clip them if necessary.

Check for objects that have been caught between pads e.g. stones, small pieces of broken glass, any other dirt or debris. Remove them, using tweezers if necessary.

Check the pads for any cuts and apply first aid if so.

Large animals

Horse and goat hooves grow very quickly. In the wild they naturally get worn down but domesticated horses normally need a professional to trim the hoof.

Check regularly for any objects stuck in the hoof and remove them.

Check for thrush - this is a strong smelling bacterial infection with black discharge. Anitbacterial treatments are available.

Birds

Bird claws continually grow and should be inspected for trimming.

The scales of the feet can become infected by mites, which causes crusty lesions to form. The mites need to be treated and the scales removed after bathing.

Mouth / dental care

Check the mucous membranes as previously described in Section 1.1 for all animals.

Dogs, cats and rodents

Check the condition of the teeth: they should be clean, in good conditon and free of discolourations.

Foul-smelling breath can be a sign of an underlying medical condition.

Ensure there is no inflammation of the gums or unusual lumps.

Rodents' teeth grow constantly and are prone to becoming overgrown, so check to see if they are protruding - if so they need clipping by a vet.

Large animals

The grinding action of horses' teeth tends to create sharp points that need removing or 'floating' by a professional.

Birds

Birds' beaks grow constantly and while this growth is normally worn down naturally, sometimes they can become overgrown. Trimming a beak should only be done by a vet.

Ear care

Dogs and cats

Check ears for dirt, debris and wax. Small amounts can be cleaned using cotton wool dipped in lukewarm water after the animal is appropriately restrained. Never insert anything directly into the ear.

Try to keep dogs' ears dry to prevent infections.

Generally little ongoing care is needed unless unusual sypmtoms are detected, in which case consult a vet.

Grooming and skin/scale care

Grooming helps to remove dead skin and improves the look and condition of a coat. It is normally pleasurable for an animal. It helps to get them used to being handled, and helps create a bond between you and the animal.

Dogs and cats

Long-haired breeds will moult as they shed their winter and summer coats; however if kept indoors with fairly constant temperatures coats may continue to moult all year round.

Whilst cats are effective self-groomers they still benefit from grooming. Long-haired varieties of cats and dogs require more regular grooming.

The grooming procedure in dogs should focus on the legs, then the tail, body, chest and head.

You can use your grooming sessions to check the other aspects of the animals' health listed here.

Large animals

Grooming is important for horses for the same reasons as for cats and dogs. It helps stimulate oils in the skin as well as removing dead skin and hair.

A detailed guide to grooming a horse goes beyond the scope of this book but includes a number of different combs and brushes.

Ideally horses would be groomed daily but certainly before and after riding.

You should be aware of the horse's reaction to your grooming, in order to inform how firmly or gently to press.

Birds

Birds do not need to be groomed but they do need access to water to bathe in.

Eyes

For all species, eyes should be bright, clear (not cloudy) and free of any discharge. If they are not then this can be a sign of infection or disease and should be referred to a vet.

Weighing

An animal's weight is one indicator of its general health. Therefore an animal should be weighed at regular intervals and records should be kept so that changes over time can be monitored and acted upon as necessary.

There are no hard and fast rules about how often different species of animal should be weighed but animals in poor health or with suspected health conditons should be weighed more often than fit and healthy animals.

Obesity is potentially fatal for animals yet is a growing problem amongst pets. If in doubt, weighing more often is preferable to weighing less often.

Species or breed-specific needs

You must be aware of particular husbandry requirements for the species you are looking after. You can use the headings in these sections to help but be aware that there might be some other category of husbandry requirements not covered here, particularly for exotic animals.

Jargon Buster

parasite organisms that obtain food from a host organism.

host organism that a parasite lives and feeds on

topical the surface of the body

oral the mouth

larvae a stage of development between birth and adults that some animals go through e.g. a caterpillar is a larval stage of a butterfly

Activity

Research some common care routines for your chosen species.

Quiz Questions

1 What is a parasite?

2 Describe the main features of a) ticks, b) lice.

3 What routine care might you give to a parrot?

LO2 Recognise how to promote and maintain the welfare of animals

2.1 Current animal welfare legislation and how these relate to health and husbandry

In this topic you will learn about the aims and purpose of the following legislation:

- **The Animal Welfare Act 2006 and Animal Health and Welfare Act (Scotland) (2006)**

- **The Animal Welfare (Licensing of Activities Involving Animals) (England) Regulations 2018**

- **The Welfare of Animal (Transport) (England) Order 2006**

- **The Dangerous Dogs Act**

- **The Veterinary Surgeons Act 1966**

- **The Welfare of Farmed Animals Regulations 2007**

- **Legislation specific to species.**

Animal welfare legislation refers to laws that exist to protect animals. You should be aware of the following, and any others that may relate to your selected species.

Animal Welfare Act 2006 and Animal Health and Welfare Act (Scotland) (2006)

Aim: To ensure all animals have all of their welfare needs met.

Purpose: To make it illegal for anyone to mistreat animals. Owners or keepers need to ensure that five animal welfare needs are met:

- have a normal diet

- are housed in a suitable environment (place to live)

- are housed with or without other animals, as is considered normal for that particular species

- are free of 'pain, injury, suffering and disease'

- exhibit behaviour that is normal for that species.

The Animal Welfare (Licensing of Activities Involving Animals) (England) Regulations 2018

Aim: To regulate and license professionals who work with animals.

Purpose: These Regulations are part of the Animal Welfare Act 2006 and provide a license scheme for the following activities:

- selling animals as pets

- breeding dogs

- catteries and dog kennels

- day care of dogs

- hiring out horses

- keeping or training animals for exhibition.

Any business that wants to conduct any of these activities requires a licence from their local authority to do so. That licence is granted if they meet five general conditions, as well as conditions specific to each activity. The general conditions are around the five welfare needs:

- need for a suitable environment
- need for a suitable diet
- need to exhbit normal behaviour patterns,
- need to be housed with or apart from other animals as appropriate
- need to be protected from pain, suffering, injury and disease.

See section 2.2 for more information on these needs.

Welfare of Animal (Transport) (England) Order 2006

Aim: To regulate how animals are transported from place to place.

Purpose: To enforce minimum requirements on the transportation of animals in line with commercial activities. This means that there are rules about the following:

- whether an animal can be transported in the first place
- how much space different animals must be given
- how long journeys can last for without a break for food and water
- provision of adequate food and water
- adequate ventilation and temperature
- provision of litter for toileting
- the transporter must be able to provide first aid.

This is not an exhaustive list. The rules are slightly different for different animals, and animal welfare must be checked throughout the journey. If animals are travelling for more than 50km then the vehicle must have an animal transport certificate that includes details about where the animals came from, are going and how long they have been travelling, amongst other things.

Dangerous Dogs Act 1991

Aim: to prevent injury and death due to aggressive or out-of-control dogs.

Purpose: this Act makes it illegal to own, sell

or breed four particular breeds of dog: the Pit Bull Terrier, the Japanese Tosa, the Dogo Argentino, and the Fila Brasiliera. (Note the Pit Bull Terrier is not to be confused with other types of bull terriers, such as Staffordshire Bull Terriers.) The Act also makes it a criminal offence for an owner to allow any breed of dog to be dangerously out of control. Such dogs may be seized by the police and ultimately destroyed.

The Veterinary Surgeons Act 1966

Aim: To regulate vets.

Purpose: This Act states that someone can only operate on animals, or call themselves a vet, if they are listed on a register of veterinary surgeons. It states the procedures on animals that non-vets are allowed to perform, and those that only vets can perform. There are some amendments to the Act that were made in 1988 and 2002.

The Welfare of Farmed Animals Regulations 2007

Aim: To implement EU regulations on the welfare of farmed livestock.

Purpose: These regulations are made under the Animal Welfare Act 2006. These regulations have been made to ensure that the Act implements all relevant EU directives on farming animals, which the UK had previously signed up to. The Regulations replace the The Welfare of Farmed Animals (England) 2000 and remove duplication that exists between the 2000 Regulations and the Animal Welfare Act 2006.

Legislation specific to species

Beyond the listed legislation there may be other pieces of legislation that are relevant to the animals or species you are working with. You should make sure you are aware of this legislation. In addition, legislation does change over time, and may be more likely to do so following the UK's departure from the EU. You should make sure you know of any upcoming changes to the list above.

1 What is the purpose of The Welfare of Animal (Transport) (England) Order 2006?

2 Give three examples of activities covered by The Animal Welfare (Licensing of Activities Involving Animals) (England) Regulations 2018?

3 Outline the main points of The Dangerous Dogs Act 1991.

2.2 Care and husbandry requirements in relation to the five welfare needs

In this topic you will learn about the:

- **Need for a suitable diet**

- **Need for a suitable environment**

- **Need to be able to exhibit normal behaviour patterns**

- **Need to be housed with, or apart, from other animals**

- **Need to be protected from pain, suffering, injury and disease.**

There are five animal welfare needs, which are defined in The Animal Welfare Act 2006. Each of these needs inform how you can properly look after that species.

Need for a suitable diet

Each species of animal needs a particular combination of nutrients in order for their body to repair itself, keep in good condition, fight off illness, have enough energy for their normal lifestyle and to generally maintain a good level of health. Most important nutrients need to provided by the food they eat.

Different species of animal need different amounts of each nutrient, and so each species needs a different diet.

Each individual animal within the same species needs different amounts of each nutrient according to it's life stage (e.g. elderly, young, pregnant) and lifestyle (e.g. active, inactive, working).

To provide a suitable diet for each individual animal you must know about and consider each of these aspects.

Need for a suitable environment

All animal species have evolved over tens or hundreds of thousands of years to adapt to their natural environment. This means that different species need different things from their environment in captivity. You should be aware of what those needs are for the species you are working with. However, all animal environments should be clean, dry (unless aquatic) and kept at the correct temperature, with access to adequate food and water, and somewhere to go to the toilet. Opportunities for exercise, play and intellectual stimulation are also necessary for many species. The environment must also be free of hazards.

Need to be able to exhibit normal behaviour patterns.

Animals must be allowed to behave in a way that is natural for the species. Animals that are prevented from doing so normally develop some behavioural or health problems.

For instance, most animals are active in the wild. Therefore, whilst in captivity, they need a certain amount of exercise to stay fit and healthy. It would be cruel to prevent active animals like dogs from exercising by not taking them for walks. Natural roamers such as cats normally need to be allowed to roam just like their ancestors and wild cousins.

Similarly, animals have evolved waking and sleeping routines that they should be allowed to follow as closely as possible. Keeping animals awake with bright lights or noise, when they would normally be sleeping, would prevent them from exhibiting their normal pattern of behaviour.

Need to be housed with, or apart, from other animals.

Innappropriate housing can result in aggression and/or mental stress. Examples of inappropriate groups include:

- naturally sociable animals being kept alone

- naturally solitary animals being kept in groups

- forcing together individual animals who, whilst sociable, are in different social groups

- incorrect social structures within social groups, for example adolescents maturing into adults that would have left the group in the wild, introduction of new animals that upset the established hierarchies

- removal of family members who are really important for the group, for example the heads of the group

- competing males and/or females during mating periods.

It may sometimes also be inappropriate for different breeds to live together.

Close proximity to other species may also cause serious stress – particular for predator and prey species. In that case stress may be induced in both the predator and the prey.

Need to be protected from pain, suffering, injury and disease

Any animal that is not in the wild is in an unnatural situation. They therefore rely on humans to protect them. Whilst they are in our care they have the right to be protected from pain and suffering, injury and disease. This means that they are not kept in such a way that might cause accidents, encourage ill-health or promote illness. Their living area must be kept free of hazards and kept clean. They must be protected from predators or aggression from other animals, and the potential for accidents should be assessed, with measures to prevent them put in place.

Behaviour such as leaving dogs in hot cars in the summer, or giving animals the wrong food as treats can all cause serious pain and suffering - even if that was not the intention.

Disregard for any of the previous welfare needs above is also likely to cause cause pain and suffering.

> **Jargon Buster**
>
> aquatic water-based.
>
> adolescent the oldest young animals.

Quiz Questions

1 Name two of the animal welfare needs.

2 Give one example of an inappropriate environment for an animal species you are studying.

3 Why does a suitable diet depend on the characteristics of the species and individual animal?

LO3 Identify signs and symptoms of common diseases and disorders, their prevention and treatment

3.1 Signs and symptoms of common diseases, their prevention and treatments

In this topic you will learn about the cause, signs, treatment and prevention of common diseases caused by the following pathogens:

- Viral: parvo, cat flu, myxomatosis, equine influenza, equine herpes virus, herpes virus, avian flu

- Bacterial: strangles, leptospirosis, salmonella, kennel cough, tetanus, white spot

- Fungal: ringworm, thrush

- Parasitic: mites, ticks, lice, fleas, gill flukes, fly strike

Viral

Disease	Signs	Treatment	Prevention
Parvovirus – different versions of this virus can affect a large range of animals but is common in dogs (canine parvovirus or CPV) and cats (feline parvovirus or FPV). It is spread by direct or indirect contact with infected animals' faeces or other bodily fluids.	Deydration, vomiting, fever, diarrhoea. The disease attacks the intestines and infected dogs and cats are likely to die.	There are no treatments for parvovirus. However an animal's immune systems can fight the disease with the aid of medical support. If an animal is suspected of parvovirus, contact a vet immediately.	Part of the standard vaccinations given to puppies and kittens. Prevention is far more effective than any other measure. Highly contagious, so strict disinfection and isolation techniques must be used following an outbreak.
Cat flu – like a human cold but caused by feline herpes virus (FHV) or feline calicivirus (FCV). Not serious for adult cats but a vet should be consulted.	Similar to a human cold - runny nose, streaming eyes, sneezing and aches and pains.	Like a human cold, a cat needs to be supported to fight off the virus. This means ensuring they are hydrated and looking out for secondary bacterial infections which might require antibiotics.	Prevention of FHC and FCV forms part of the standard vaccinations given to kittens. .

Disease	Signs	Treatment	Prevention
Myxomatosis – a disease that affects rabbits. It is a very serious condition that is almost always fatal. It is common in wild rabbits and can spread through insect bites or direct contact.	Swollen, weeping or milky eyes, swelling of face and genital area, scabs around the body, high temperature, lack of appetite.	Unvaccinated rabbits are unlikely to survive. Vaccinated rabbits stand a better chance but would still require intensive care from a vet.	Prevention is by far best option. There is a standard vaccination for pet rabbits but preventing infection is equally important. This means keeping living areas clean, treating your rabbit and other animals for fleas, and preventing contact with wild rabbits.
Equine influenza - also known as horse flu, this is a very contagious respiratory disease. It is not normally fatal.	Coughing, discharge from the nose, high temperature.	Like human flu, treatment is mainly limited to rest, and ensuring the horse is well fed and watered. If secondary infections occur then separate treatment may be needed for those.	Standard annual vaccinations are available.
Equine herpes has two main strains that cause problems - a respiratory version which leads to breathing problems and a neurological version, which affects the brain and can cause paralysis and abortion in pregnant mares.	Coughing, discharge from the nose, high temperature. The strain that affects the brain also has symtptoms that affect the coordination of limbs.	Like equine influenza, most horses will recover and simply need rest and care.	Standard vaccinations are available for the respiratory strain. Infected horses should be isolated from other horses, and strict infection control put in place as the virus is very infectious.
Herpes is the name for a wide family of viruses that infects animals and humans. Specifc strains normally infect specific species, e.g. feline herpes virus (FHV) and canine herpes virus (CHV). CHV is particularly dangerous for puppies - most puppies will die if they catch it.	For puppies, CHV is accompanied by general weakness, a lack of suckle reflex and crying. For cats, FHV is a disease of the respiratory tract and eyes, with symptoms such as coughing, sneezing, nasal discharge and conjunctivitis (build up of deposits on the eyelid.)	There are no successful treatments for puppies with CHV. Cats with FHV will be treated according to their symptoms until they are better.	There is a standard vaccine for FHV. There is a non-standard vacccine for CHV, which has to be administered to mothers, who can then pass on their antibodies to her puppies. The best prevention strategy, however, is to avoid contact between a heavily pregnant bitch/ puppies with infected dogs. However a large number of adult dogs do carry the disease so this can be quite difficult.

Disease	Signs	Treatment	Prevention
Avian flu – also known as 'bird flu', this virus is transmitted by direct contact between birds or through bodily fluids and faeces. It is not an airborne disease.	Swollen head, breathing problems, coughing, sneezing, blue tinge to head, diarrhoea, reduced appetite, fewer laid eggs.	There are two versions of avian flu – birds with the less serious version will normally get better by themselves but the more serious version is deadly and there is currently no known cure.	Vaccines have been developed but their effectiveness is uncertain. Avian flu is highly infectious so the best prevention is to prevent contact with infected birds, particularly wild birds. Any birds with symptoms should be isolated immediately, and the area cleaned and disinfected.

Bacterial

Disease	Signs	Treatment	Prevention
Strangles - a disease of the upper respiratory tract that affects horses.	High temperature, lack of appetite, yellow nasal discharge, enlarged lymph nodes.	Antibiotics.	A standard vaccination is available. But any horse with an uncertain health history should be isolated for a time until it is sure they do not have strangles.
Salmonella – a bacterial infection of the intestine that many animals carry without becoming ill. The bacteria can be passed on to unborn animals from their mother, or by direct contact. The bacteria are present in faeces and can then contaminate the environment. In addition it can be spread through eating contaminated meat or animal products.	Many animals naturally have the bacteria and are not ill. But animals that do get ill have symptoms such as diarrhoea, vomiting, fever and loss of appetite.	Antibiotics, and ensuring the animal is sufficiently hydrated.	Keeping animals' living areas clean, and cleaning up animal faeces, will help prevent transmission between animals. Humans should thoroughly wash their hands after touching animals to avoid contracting the disease. Particularly careful hygiene procedures should be put in place when handlng exotic species as they can carry the disease.

Disease	Signs	Treatment	Prevention
Leptospirosis – a bacterial disease spread through the urine of animals, often passed on through contaminated water.	Vomiting, fever, abdominal pain, diarrhoea, weakness, loss of appetite.	Antibiotics.	Rodents such as rats and mice are often responsible for infection, so limiting exposure to them helps prevent the disease. Ensruing food storage is completely free of vermin. Vaccinations are also available though are not always 100% effective.
Kennel cough - an infectious respiratory conditon in dogs that causes a swollen windpipe and larynx. It is caused by the bacteria **Bordetella bronchiseptica**	A persistent and distinctive cough and nasal discharge.	Antibiotics are available but otherwise fit and healthy dogs normally recover naturally with rest and care.	Standard vaccination available. Very contagious, so easily spreads when dogs are kept together - hence the name. Dogs suspected of the condition should be separated from other dogs.
Tetanus - an infection caused by bacteria that lives in soil, normally transmitted through infected wounds. It causes muscle spasms (and is also known as 'lock-jaw'). Horses are particularly susceptible.	Standing rigidly, difficulty walking and turning, patches of sweat. Severe cases can cause death as animals struggle to breathe.	Antibiotics to kill the bacteria and sedatives to help with the muscle spasms.	A vaccine is available and is a standard vaccine for horses.
White spot - a disease, caused by a parasite, which affects fish and is also known as **Ichthyophthirius multifiliis** or Ich	Appearance of small white spots on the body of fish caused by the burrowing of the parasite. If left untreated white spot can kill.	Chemicals can be added to water that kill the parasite.	Quarantine new fish for a couple of weeks before introducing to other fish. Water should be kept clean.

Fungal

Disease	Signs	Treatment	Prevention
Thrush – a yeast that can infect different parts of the body (ear, mouth, skin) and different animals.	It depends on where the infection takes hold - scratching if on the skin, drooling if in the mouth.	Antifungal medication.	Thrives in damp and dirty conditions. Targets animals with weakened immune systems. So good diet and cleanliness is key.
Ringworm – not a worm but a fungus which lives in the top layer of the skin and in hair follicles, and is spread through direct contact. It is not life-threatening.	Circular patches (which give the disease its name), red and scabby skin, patches of hair or fur loss, dry and brittle coat, brittle claws.	Topical treatments (creams, shampoo, ointments) and anti-fungal oral medication. Cleaning and treatment of the animal's environment to remove infected hair.	Keeping the environment clean is the main preventative measure. Vaccines are available e.g. Ringvac.

Parasitic

Disease	Signs	Treatment	Prevention
Mites - tiny animals of less than 1mm, that feed on dead skin or the host's blood.	Itching, skin irritation, sore or dry skin, poor skin conditon, dark crusts of skin in the ears.	Sprays, powders, dips and shampoos.	Separate infected animals, and keep living and bedding areas clean.
Ticks - around 3-5mm in size, they move from one host to another and feed off each of the host's blood. Ticks can carry other diseases, most notably Lyme disease.	Itching, skin irritation, fur loss, dull coat. Other symptoms might occur due to disease caused by ticks.	Sprays, powders, tablets, collars and shampoos.	Higher-risk environments include wooded and vegetated areas, so keeping an animal indoors or restricting their movement when outside can help prevent ticks.
Lice - under 5mm long, there are two different types of lice - biting lice (that live off dead skin/hair/feathers) and blood-sucking lice (that feed off their host's blood).	Itching, poor skin condition, loss of hair or fur, sight of the lice or their eggs (known as nits).	Sprays, shampoos, powders will kill the lice. However the nits are unaffected, and so treatment should continue until all nits have hatched.	Lice can only survive on the host species, so infected animals should be separated until treated. All bedding, combs etc. should not be shared and thoroughly disinfected.

Disease	Signs	Treatment	Prevention
Fleas - around 3mm in length, fleas live on a host's skin and feed on their blood.	Skin irritation and 'flea dirt' - tiny dark specks of digested blood that a flea has excreted can be combed out of an animal's fur. Very common in dogs.	Using sprays, powders, tablets and shampoos, as well as removing flea eggs through vaccuming and disinfecting bedding and living areas.	Flea treatments in tablet or other forms are available to prevent fleas.
Gill flukes - around 3mm or smaller, these parasites lodge themselves in the gills of a fish to feed on skin.	Fish rising to the surface of the water to try and breathe, mucuous forming around the gills, inflammation of gills.	Quarantine the affected fish and then treat the quarantined tank with commercially available gill fluke treatments.	Quarantine new fish and plants for 2 weeks before introducing to main environment, and regularly clean and refresh water.
Fly strike - an infestation of maggots, hatched from eggs laid by flies, that feed on the host's dead flesh. This is a serious condition that can result in death. Suspected cases should be reported to a vet immediately.	Flies are more likely to lay eggs on animals with open wounds and animals that are ill, dirty, or unable to clean themselves. You may see small larvae and there may be a foul smell. The animal may display signs of skin irritation.	The maggots need to be physically removed, dead skin cut away and the wound area fully cleaned and disinfected.	Fly strike is more common in warm weather when there are more flies around. In these months animals should be kept clean and wounds protected if they are likely to come into contact with flies.

Jargon Buster

virus genetic material which invades cells in the body and takes over their ability to replicate in order to make copies of the virus instead. Viruses are very, very small - a million times smaller than a millimetre and a thousand times smaller than bacteria, which means that some viruses can even infect bacteria!

bacteria single-celled organisms, they are a thousand times smaller than a millimetre.

fungus can be single-celled or made of multiple cells, with a huge variety of size and structure. Some fungus are tiny whilst others can easily be seen with the naked eye - for example, mushrooms are a type of fungus.

parasite any organism that lives and feeds on another organism such as a plant or animal.

intestine organs of the digestive system in the body

respiratory relating to breathing

Quiz Questions

1 List three bacterial diseases.

2 Describe the signs and treatment of two viruses that particularly affect cats.

3 List two diseases that specifically affect horses.

4 Describe the differences between a flea and a tick.

3.2 Common disorders, their signs and treatments

In this topic you will learn about common physical medical and behavioural disorders:

- **Medical: Metabolic Bone Disease, Cushing's syndrome, Epilepsy, Arthritis**

- **Behavioural: Stress and anxiety, Feather plucking, Obesity, Pica, Over grooming**

These disorders are caused by influencing factors:

- **Lack of appropriate stimulation**

- **Exercise**

- **Socialisation, companionship, separation and social factors**

- **Poor handling**

- **Inadequate diet (diabetes, obesity, gut stasis)**

- **Inappropriate accommodation**

Whilst the previous section covered diseases, there are also a range of disorders that affect animals - both physical and behavioural. Such disorders can be influenced by the following factors described below. You will be expected to know about the common physical and behavioural disorders, as described in this section, for a minimum of two species from the range that was described at the start of the unit.

Lack of appropriate stimulation

Animals in the wild do not have anyone to feed them or look after them. They commonly need to solve problems in order to find food and shelter, and their brains have evolved in order to do so. Their environment also provides lots of stimulation - different shapes, objects and other animals.

In captivity, animals no longer have to find their own food and may live in an environment that doesn't change. This means they no longer have the mental stimulation that their brains have evolved to cope with. This can lead them to them becoming bored. To recreate the wild, animals can be mentally stimulated by games, puzzles, or encouraging

them to forage for food.

Exercise

Different animal species are different shapes and sizes, have different nutritional needs and eat different types, and amounts, of food. They also all need different amounts of exercise to be fit and healthy. Over-exercise places too much stress on the body and can lead to physical injuries. Under-exercise can cause a number of issues, which we will discuss shortly.

Socialisation, companionship, separation and social factors

Different species naturally behave in different ways with other animals:

- Some animals are very sociable and will always live together in groups in the wild.

- Other animals are very solitary in the wild and rarely interact with other animals.

- Some social animals have complex rules regarding the members of the group.

This general behaviour may also change at

different points in an animal's life.

Forcing solitary animals together, or separating sociable animals, can lead to abnormal behaviour, aggression and mental stress.

Poor handling

Animals in captivity will have contact with and be handled by humans throughout their lives. This might be for medical reasons, for transportation or as part of normal health-checking routines.

Animals that have been used to being handled in an appropriate fashion from a young age are likely to be able to tolerate considerate handling throughout their lives. Animals that are unused to be being handled, or were treated poorly by previous handlers, may display signs of nervousness, aggression, hostility or fear.

Inadequate diet

Animals' bodies need a complex combination of nutrients in order to correctly function. These nutrients are normally obtained through their diet. Different food types have different quantities of nutrients and a balanced diet for an animal will ensure that they receive nutrients in the correct quantities. However, because each species has different nutritional requirements a balanced diet for one species is not necessarily a balanced diet for another. Animals of the same species can also have different nutritional requirements, depending on age, lifestyle, medical conditions and so on.

There are many potential implications of a inadequate diet - i.e. one containing incorrect quantities of nutrients for that animal. Some common ones are:

- **Diabetes** - this is a condition where insulin in the body cannot be produced in sufficient quantities, or the body responds inadequately to it. Insulin is critical to the conversion of food into energy. Diabetes can be caused by a diet containing too much fat and carbohydrate. Obese animals are more at risk of diabetes.

- **Obesity** - this is when animals are overweight and have an excess of body fat. It carries serious health risks and can

be caused by a diet that contains more energy than the animal needs. This excess energy is stored in the form of body fat.

- **Gut stasis** - common in rabbits and guinea pigs, this is when the normal movement of food through the digestive organs slows down or stops. This can cause dehydration and malnutrition and can kill. It can be caused by a diet that is low in fibre.

Inappropriate accommodation

Any accommodation for an animal is unnatural. However the aim should always be for accommodation to meet all of the needs of the animal. In practice this means:

- Allowing an animal enough space to roam, in accordance with its behaviour in the wild.

- Ensuring that the environment is clean, dry and at the correct temperature according to the animal's needs.

- Ensuring access to adequate food, a constant supply of clean water, and somewhere to go the toilet.

- Providing opportunities for exercise, play and intellectual stimulation.

- Ensuring that noise and light levels are appropiate at different times of the day.

It goes without saying that the environment should also be free of hazards. The presence of other animals nearby should also be considered, as this can be a source of anxiety - for instance, predators housed next to prey can cause both animals considerable stress.

Behavioural disorders

Disorder	Causes	Signs	Treatment and Prevention
Stress and anxiety	There are many potential causes, including the factors previously listed: lack of stimulation, socialisation issues, poor handling, inappropriate accommodation.	As well as the disorders below, stress may show up through meaningless repetition (pacing up and down, rocking side to side), excessive scratching or touching, excessive sleeping, general disinterest, any unusual behaviour.	The cause of any stress must be identified in order to treat it. Ensuring the animal feels safe and comfortable is of course very important. A consultation with a vet is helpful.
Feather plucking - a conditon that is only really seen in captivity.	Normally in response to stress. This might be brought on by lack of stimulation, separation, poor handling, inappropriate accommodation.	Chewing or plucking of feathers.	Remove any sources of stress and consult a vet.
Obesity - excessive weight that hinders the animal's quality of life. It has serious negative health consequences.	Lack of exercise, inappropriate diet, age; occasionally a sign of disease or illness,	Visibly overweight with excess body fat, cannot or will not exercise.	A combination of diet and exercise, after consultation with a vet.
Pica - eating non-edible objects or material. This can have serious consequences for health.	Stress, lack of stimulation, separation, poor diet (malnutrition). Can also be caused by some diseases.	Vomiting, diarrhoea, constipation, witnessing an animal eating objects such as faeces, rocks, soil, paper etc.	Removing the causes, keeping the animal away from non-food objects, exercise, dietary changes.
Over grooming - excessive self-cleaning.	It might be due to skin conditions (in order scratch an itch or relieve pain), or it might be due to stress - the act of grooming is comforting to an animal.	Bald patches, broken skin, poor quality coat.	Remove the source of anxiety, or treat the skin condition.

Medical disorders

Disorder	Causes	Signs	Treatment and Prevention
Metabolic Bone Disease - a broad term for a range of diseases that affect bone strength.	Inadequate diet - deficiency of certain minerals such as phosphorus and calcium in the diet.	More common in exotic animals such as reptiles, signs include bowed legs, bumps on the bones of the leg and an arched spine.	A suitable diet will treat and prevent the condition.
Cushing's syndrome - excessive production of a stress hormone called cortisol. This leads to a weakened immune system which can lead to lots of further problems.	Abnormal functioning of the adrenal glands or pituitary glands, normally caused by a tumour.	Bloated stomach, hair loss, increased thirst and appetite, lethargy.	Most animals require medication for the rest of their life to when diagnosed, though a small number can be cured through surgery to remove the tumour.
Epilepsy - abnormal electrical signal activity in the brain.	Often inherited in dogs.	Fits and seizures, excessive salivation. completely rigid body or other unusual physical behaviour.	Antiepilepsy drugs.
Arthritis - unusual wearing of the cartilage in joints, that leads to bones rubbing against each other. Very painful condition.	Lack of exercise or a poor diet - overweight animals are more at risk. The condition normally reveals itself in older animals, once cartilage has worn away. Some breeds of animals may be more likely to develop it.	Limping or other unusual movement, general mobility issues.	Ensure animals are at a healthy weight throughout their life. Anti-inflammatory drugs and special diets can help animals who have developed the condition.

Jargon Buster
hormone a chemical in the body that send signals from the brain to different parts of the body.

Quiz Questions

1 List two behavioural disorders and two medical disorders.

2 What disorders might be caused by an inadequate diet?

3 What factors might lead to a dog developing arthritis?

4 What factors might contribute to stress in an animal?

LO4 Understand the practices and principles of animal first aid

4.1 The contents of an animal first aid box

In this topic you will learn about:

• The typical items in a first aid box

First Aid box contents

Selection of bandages, adhesive tape
Used to dress wounds and keep them clean.

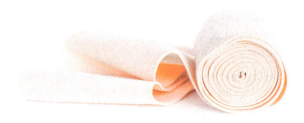

Figure 6 A bandage

Cotton wool, sterile dressing materials
Cotton wool can be used for padding and dressing material is used on the site of a wound.

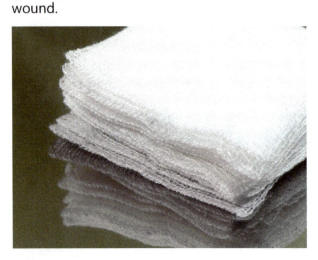

Figure 7 Dressing material

Tweezers
Used to remove thorns, splinters, stings.

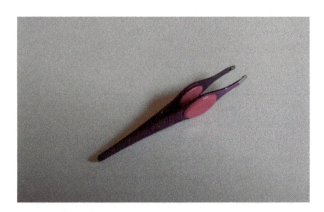

Figure 8 Tweezers

Gloves, hand sanitiser
Used to prevent cross-contamination and for protection against infections and chemicals used in treatments/medicines.

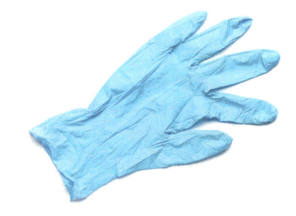

Figure 9 Gloves

Scissors

For cutting bandages, tape, dressing material or fur.

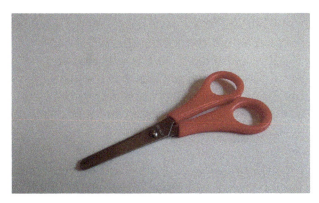

Figure 10 Scissors

Eye wash, antiseptic solution

In case of debris in the eye.

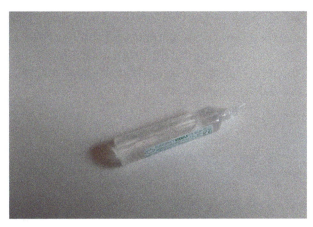

Figure 11 Eye-wash

Contact details for the local veterinary practice

Vital in an emergency.

Carrier bag, foil blanket

To help keep animals warm after an incident but can also be used as a makeshift stretcher.

Poultice

A soft moist compound that is applied to the skin to draw out infections. These are commercially available.

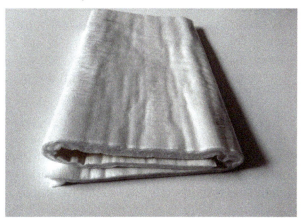

Figure 12 A poultice

Topical treatment for bites and stings

Creams and ointments to be applied to the skin.

4.2 The main principles of animal first aid

In this topic you will learn about the main principles of first aid:

- **The three aims: preserve life, prevent suffering, prevent situation deteriorating**

- **The four rules: assess situation, maintain airway, control bleeding and get help**

First aid is the immediate help and care given to an acutely ill or injured animal.

The three aims of animal first aid are to:

- preserve life
- prevent suffering
- prevent the situation from deteriorating.

In extreme cases, providing the correct care quickly can mean the difference between life and death, or a full and partial recovery. There are four rules that you must follow when carrying out first aid:

Assess situation

If you are confronted with a first aid situation, you need to assess if it is a minor, immediate or life-threatening situation. Life-threatening situations clearly need immediate action. However, in all cases you should:

- Stay calm.

- Ensure you are not putting yourself or others at further risk before taking any action.

Be aware that animals in pain or distress may be aggressive towards you or others, which may cause you an injury and further harm the animal. This is the case even for animals that are normally very friendly and docile. You will need to consider restraining and/or muzzling before handling.

When assessing or examining an animal you will need to stay very calm - remember the animal is likely to be frightened. You can try to soothe them as much as possible by talking quietly and reassuringly, and being careful to make no sudden movements. You should try not to touch or move the animal unless it is strictly necessary.

Maintain airway

An animal that cannot breathe will die in a matter of minutes. So it is vital that you ensure their airway is clear, and they can breathe, throughout the first aid procedure. Remember that the tongue can block the airway.

Control bleeding

An animal that is bleeding heavily is at risk of death. Any visible bleeding should be stopped or reduced as soon as possible.

Get help

When performing first aid you are trying to stabilise the animal so that you can get help. The sooner you get help from a veterinary surgeon the better the likely outcome for the animal concerned.

Quiz Questions

1 List three items you would expect to see in a first aid box.

2 What is a poultice and when might it be used?

3 What are the three aims of first aid?

4 If you witnessed a cat being run over, what is the first thing you should do?

4.3 Assist in first aid procedures for common animal injuries and ailments

In this topic you will learn about assisting in the assessment of an animal's overall needs/ conditions requiring first aid:

- **Recognition of limitations of responsibility and when to call for help**

- **Legal restrictions when administering first aid under the Veterinary Surgeons Act (1966)**

- **Methods to maintain human health and safety**

- **Maintenance of the airway and monitoring breathing**

- **Treatment for bleeding, including cleaning wounds**

- **Monitor pulse/circulation**

- **Temperature regulation in relation to shock**

- **Transportation/ moving of the injured animal**

- **Report to vet and or local authority if necessary**

- **Response of the animal, records of the injury, reporting to the vet/owner**

Common first aid injuries and ailments as appropriate to species:

- **Shock, wounds/bleeding, hoof injuries, colic, hypothermia, hyperthermia, convulsions, choking, poisoning, burns and scalds, bites and stings**

Recognition of limitations of responsibility and when to call for help

First aid is limited to the three aims that have been stated. This means ensuring the best possible outcome for the animal whilst keeping yourself, others and the animal safe. Where medical assistance is required, you must get full medical help from a veterinary surgeon as soon as possible.

First aid does not involve diagnosing what might be the cause of any illness or condition.

Legal restrictions when administering first aid under the Veterinary Surgeons Act (1966)

This Act states that someone can only operate on animals, or call themselves a vet, if they are listed on a register of veterinary surgeons. It states the procedures on animals that non-vets are allowed to perform, and those that only vets can perform.

Therefore, when giving first aid, it must be remembered that it is illegal for anyone other than a vet to perform medical procedures on an animal. First aid must be limited to the three aims outlined.

Methods to maintain human health and safety

There may be a number of hazards present in a first aid situation.

- An animal in pain may injure a human if not suitably restrained.

- The situation itself may be hazardous - for instance a road traffic accident. Treating an animal on a busy road may put your life in danger, or the lives of others who are using the road.

The risk to human health and safety must be assessed before any first aid action is taken.

Maintenance of the airway and monitor breathing

The first priority must be to ensure the animal can breathe. As well as clearing any obstructions, you should also monitor breathing as treatment is taking place, to ensure it does not stop.

Treatment for bleeding, including cleaning wounds

An animal's life is in danger if it is losing a lot of blood, so heavy bleeding needs to be stopped or reduced.

See the next section for details of this and cleaning wounds.

Monitor pulse/circulation

An animal's pulse is a measure of how well its heart is pumping blood around the body. A weak pulse, or no pulse at all, is very serious as it means there is a problem with their heart and oxygen is not being fully transported around the body. This can quickly lead to death.

If this is the case it may be possible to perform CPR (cardio pulmonary resuscitation).

Temperature regulation in relation to shock

Body heat should be conserved in an animal suffering from shock - this might be as simple as wrapping them in a blanket. You should not attempt to heat the animal up, however. Further details about shock follow on the next page.

Transportation and moving the injured animal

You should aim to move an injured animal as little as possible. If you do need to move them, for instance to keep them away from a hazard or take them to a vet, then get someone to help if at all possible.

- You can use a blanket for a makeshift stretcher, or even the parcel shelf from a car.

- You could wrap a smaller animal in a towel to prevent excessive movement.

- Take particular care of animals with suspected broken bones. If there is any suspected spinal or neck injury then the animal may need to be fully restrained before moving.

Report to vet and or local authority if necessary

All but the most minor accidents and injuries will need some veterinary care. Therefore you should contact a vet as soon as possible so that they can give you the correct advice on the animal's condition. For serious injuries this is of course even more important. Road traffic accidents involving animals should be reported to the local authority.

Response of the animal, records of the injury, reporting to the vet / owner

A vet will need as much information as possible to make a judgement about what to do and when.

They will need to know how the animal is responding. As animals cannot tell us how they feel, we need to use their actions and reactions to inform us instead. This might include observations such as:

- are they unconscious or drowsy/dazed?

- how are they behaving - do they appear more fearful, aggressive, passive than normal?

- how well are they breathing?

- how well are they moving - are they limping or moving unusually?

- are they exhibiting any signs of pain?

- are they bleeding?

- what is their temperature?

- what is their pulse rate?

There may be multiple observations at different times in the first aid process.

A careful record should be kept, giving details

of what the injury was, how it occured and the observable symptoms. These details should be communicated to the vet and, where applicable, the owner.

Common first aid injuries and ailments as appropriate to species

Shock

Shock is a lack of blood supply to the major organs and/or brain. It can be triggered by a range of events but it is more than simply 'being shocked'. It is a life-threatening condition and needs to be treated immediately. Symptoms include white gums, a faint quick heartbeat, quick breaths, being cold to the touch, and a slow capillary refill time.

There are different stages and severities of shock and the aim with first aid is to prevent the condition escalating to the next more serious stage. Treatment normally includes:

- keeping the animal warm
- preventing any blood loss
- keeping airways clear
- stopping the animal from moving around
- keeping the head lower than the body.

Wounds and bleeding

If there is an open wound (i.e. the skin is broken) and it is still bleeding, cover with a dressing material and apply pressure until the bleeding stops. Do not remove the dressing once the bleeding has stopped. Ensure that there are no objects in the wound before applying pressure.

Haemorrhages – heavy bleeding – is dangerous because an animal can lose a lot of blood quickly. This can lead to shock, or it can lead to tissue damage. If it is external then heavy bleeding is obvious; but there might be internal bleeding which is not obvious. Symptoms of non-visible bleeding are:

- pale gums
- rapid pulse and/or breath

- slow capillary refill time
- coughing up blood, or blood present in the faeces.

For heavy external bleeding the main aim is to reduce or stop the bleeding:

- place a clean absorbent dressing material onto the affected point
- make sure there are no foreign objects in the wound
- press firmly on the dressing with your fingers for up to 10 minutes.

Alternatively, or additionally, you could apply a tourniquet (also known as a pressure bandage) to constrict the flow of blood to the affected area. The tourniquet can be left in place for 15 minutes.

Another alternative is to locate the nearest artery that supplies the affected area and apply pressure there to slow or stop blood flowing to the affected area.

Restricting blood flow in any of these ways is only a temporary measure because a lack of blood to the tissues will cause long-term problems - so you should consult a vet immediately in all cases of heavy bleeding.

If the open wound is minor and not bleeding, clean the wound using an antiseptic and then dress and cover.

Closed wounds are when the skin has not been broken but there is damage to the tissue underneath. Treatment aims to prevent further tissue damage. This can be done using a cold compress, by applying ice wrapped in a towel to the affected area.

Hoof injuries - abscess

A hoof abscess is caused by bacteria getting trapped inside the hoof. This may be due to an object (such as glass) causing a wound, or poor hoof care. If you see such an object you should not remove it - instead get advice from your vet. The abscess itself is build-up of fluid that causes pressure and results in a painful swelling. A hoofed animal that suddenly develops lameness, swelling or a raised temperature is likely to have developed an abscess.

To relieve symptoms of an abscess a vet will drain it of fluid. However this is something that only a vet should do. Once drained, a poultice can be applied to draw out any remaining fluid.

Colic

Colic is another name for abdominal pain and is common in horses. The cause of abdominal pain can be quite wide-ranging - from a build-up of gas in the stomach to inflammation of the intestines. Symptoms of colic include lack of interest in food, a bloated stomach, bending the head towards the torso and lying down more often than ususal.

Because there are many different causes of colic, and some are life-threatening, an animal with suspected colic should be referred to a vet as soon as possible.

Hypothermia

Animals suffering from hypothermia have a dangerously low body temperature. This temperature differs across species but both warm-blooded and cold-blooded animals will suffer if they get too cold. It is normally due to exposure to cold conditions for too long, or exposure to sudden very cold conditions. Wet animals in cold conditions can cool down very quickly. Even animals with thick coats can get hypothermia if exposed to very cold conditions.

Signs of hypothermia include shivering, pale gums, clumsy movements, tiredness and passing out.

Hypothermia is life-threatening and action must be taken immediately for any animal suspected of suffering it. You can try and warm them up very slowly and carefully - perhaps by wrapping them in a blanket. You can cause further damage if you warm them up too quickly. You must call a vet as soon as possible.

Hyperthermia

Hyperthermia is when an animal's body becomes overheated. It can be caused by a fever (i.e. an animal's temperature increases when fighting off a virus) or by environmental factors. It is very dangerous for an animal to become too hot, as it can lead to organ failure.

Signs of hyperthermia include panting, signs of dehydration, very red gums, increased heart rate, clumsy movements.

Hyperthermia is life-threatening and you must treat it as soon as possible. You can try and cool an animal down by removing them from the source of the heat, by spraying them with cool water or by placing them in water. You must not use cold water or ice - this is very dangerous as it can reduce the size of blood vessels as the surface of the skin, which will actually prevent cooling. You must also call a vet as soon as possible.

Convulsions

Also known as 'fits' or 'seizures', these result from abnormal electrical activity in the brain which interferes with the normal processes. There can be many different reasons for the abnormal activity but it will result in a lack of control of the muscles. This might mean the animal goes quite still and can't seem to move, or might lead to wild and uncontrolled movements.

- The main danger to the animal is that they hurt themselves whilst they are having a convulsion. So move any object out of the way that may provide a danger. If possible wrap the animal in a blanket.

- Keep noise to a minimum.

- Try not to touch the animal.

- Do not put anything near the animal's mouth and do not attempt to give them food or water.

- If the seizure lasts for more than a few minutes then call a vet.

Choking

An animal can only survive for a matter of minutes if unable to breathe, so immediate action needs to be taken for animals that are choking.

- Restrain the animal and check the airway for any obvious blockages (including the tongue).

- If the blockage does not come out then you can grasp both hands just below the rib cage and pull them sharply towards you. This has the affect of expelling breath, which can dislodge the object. You must be very careful, particularly with smaller animals, as the wrong hand position can break bones.

Poisoning

Animals can be poisoned through eating or breathing in a toxic substance, or through exposure to the skin. If you think an animal has been poisoned then the first thing is to establish what the poison is. Remember that poison means any substance that is toxic for an animal – this can include everyday items such as chocolate, raisins and houseplants.

Some symptoms of poisoning are:

- stomach pain
- unsteady on the feet
- salivating, vomiting
- slow capillary refill time.

If an animal has been exposed or eaten something poisonous then take action immediately – don't wait for symptoms to appear.

- Do not induce vomiting.
- Keep the animal warm and comfortable.
- Place in the recovery position.
- Note down the likely source of the poison if known.
- Get them to a vet immediately.

Burns and scalds

Burns can range from first degree (mild) to third degree (severe). A vet will need to be consulted for second and third degree burns. But for all burns you should:

- restrain the animal
- cool the area by applying a cloth soaked in cold water
- do not apply any creams or ointments
- do not break any blisters
- see a vet immediately for second and third degree burns.

Bites and stings

Bites normally result in open wounds where there is a risk of infection. Refer to the guidelines for open wounds.

Stings from insects can be painful and result in red, itchy and swollen skin.

- If the sting is still in the animal then try and remove it, taking care not to break it.
- Apply ice or a cold compress to the sting, for pain relief.

Jargon Buster
haemorrhage heavy bleeding

tourniquet something which reduces blood flow

hypothermia dangerously low body temperature

hyperthermia dangerously high body temperature

Quiz Questions

1 What are the legal restrictions with regard to performing first aid?

2 What you should you do if you suspect an animal has been poisoned?

3 Describe the main symptoms of shock.

4 For what kind of burns must you consult a vet?

5 Why can it be dangerous to leave a dog unattended in a car on a warm day?

Unit 202 Animal feeding and accommodation

LO1 Prepare equipment, food and water for animals

1.1 Prepare food and water for animals

In this topic you will learn about the different types of food:

- fresh
- dried

- tinned
- frozen

You will also learn about:

- quality of feed and longevity (shelf life)
- nutrient requirements
- dietary requirements

- number and frequency of feeds
- correct storage.

Different types of food available to selected species

Fresh

This means food that has not been processed or preserved in any way. Fresh food that has been picked will not keep and cannot be stored for very long.

- Fruit and vegetables: low in fat, low in salt, low in calories, and a good source of vitamins, minerals and fibre.

- Grass and foraged food: some animals have special digestive processes that use bacteria to break down grass and other plant material and obtain nutrients from it. For those animals grass provides energy from carbohydrates, as well as protein, fibre and minerals. Grass is a natural source of food for a number of livestock animals, and given a choice animals would normally prefer grass over hay, which is a dried food. Grass is also

cheaper than processed food. However there are reasons why hay might be a preferred food source (see next section). Because foraged food is still growing until the animal eats it, there are no issues regarding storage or the food spoiling. However foraged food may be seasonal, meaning that animals can only find it at certain times of the year.

- Fresh meat: carnivores such as cats require meat for some essential nutrients. Meat is an excellent source of protein but contains no carbohydrates. It is a source of energy however because of the relatively high fat content. Red meat and pork have high levels of fat whereas lean chicken has low levels of fat. Red meat is also a good source of vitamins and minerals.

Dried food

As the name suggests, dry food has had moisture removed from it.

Fresh food decays because microorganisms such as bacteria break it down. As part of that process they need to use the water contained in fresh food. By removing water, the decay process in dried food is dramatically slowed down.

Dried animal food might be in the form of pellets or biscuits and is convenient to store as it keeps for a long time. It also tends to be better for animals' teeth than wet food. Dry food will tend to contain more carbohydrates, derived from cereals, than fresh or tinned food.

Because there is less water present, animals on a dry food diet must be given an adequate supply of drinking water.

Concentrates

Concentrates refers to food that has high amounts of particular nutrients, such as fat, carbohydrates or protein. Dried concentrates are often in the form of pellets.

Complete food

Dried food may be processed so that it contains all of the nutrients and minerals that particular animal species needs. These complete foods are very convenient. However it must be remembered that some animals may have specific dietary needs based on their lifestyle, so even complete foods may sometimes need to be supplemented.

Preserved forages

Another common dried food is hay, which is essentially dried grass. In the drying process the grass loses moisture but also loses nutrients, and can be harder to digest. Hay is more expensive than grass, but it keeps for much longer and is often used when fresh grass is not available, for instance in winter.

Haylage is similar to hay but is formed using younger grass which is cut earlier, and then stored using a different process, called fermentation, to prevent decay. All of this leads to it having a greater moisture content than hay.

Silage is very similar to haylage but with even less moisture removed.

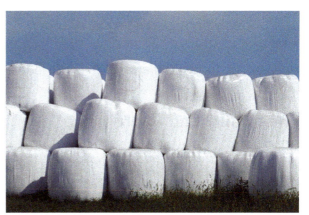
Figure 13 Haylage fermenting in a field

Tinned food

Food can be preserved by storing it in tins (or cans). The 'canning' process involves heating the tins to very high temperatures to kill off all the microorganisms, and then the air-tight tins prevent new microooganisms from spoiling the food. Whilst some nutrients are affected by this process, most are not and this ensures that nutritious food can be stored for a very long time. The process is a convenient way for meat and fish to be preserved, which is very important for animals that require them in their diet.

Wet food stored in tins or cans tends to be more expensive than dry food. With fewer carbohydrates and therefore more protein and fat, animals may prefer the taste and smell of wet food.

Food will of course spoil once tins are opened and the food is served.

Frozen

Another method to preserve food is through the freezing process. This turns the water that is present in most food into ice, which prevents the activity of the microorganisms that cause food to rot. The microogranisms are not killed however and so still pose a danger once frozen food has thawed.

Freezing preseves most of the nutritional content present when the food was frozen. So if food such as vegetables are frozen immediately after picking then they remain highly nutritious.

Water expands when frozen as ice, which

causes cells in delicate food such as fruit to break. This means that the texture of some food is not as good after freezing.

Once frozen food has thawed it must never be refrozen.

The quality and appropriate amount of feed

Quality of feed

The quality of food is really a measure of how nutritionally valuable it is; a low-quality feed, for instance, would have low levels of essential nutrients and might require supplements, or need to be fed in large volumes. Conversely a high-quality feed would provide all of the nutrients necessary for that species. Note that, because different species have different nutritional needs, what is high-quality for one species may be low-quality for another. Unsurprisingly, a low-quality feed would normally be cheaper than a high-quality one.

The appropriate amount of feed depends on the nutritional needs of the animal in question.

For commercially available feed the manufacturer will provide detailed and accurate nutritional information. However, for home-made diets or ingredients, for farmers who let livestock graze, or who grow crops for feeding animals, some method of assessing nutrition will be needed.

Nutritional information is available online for common foodstuffs and crops. A good resource to consider is www.feedipedia.org Such websites can be used as a guide when assessing home-made diets. However the exact nutritional composition of a particular crop will depend on the growing conditions, soil, climate etc. So it is important that careful monitoring of feeding takes place, to make sure that its impact on animal behaviour or output is observed.

Shelf life, longevity and best before food dates

All food has a certain shelf life, which is how long it will keep for. This is also known as its longevity. There is normally a trade-off

between quality and shelf life. Fresh food tends to be of the highest quality but will not keep for long. Foods that have been processed so that they keep for longer - such as dried food - will often have a lower nutritional quality.

Best before dates are included on the packaging of commercially available pre-prepared food, to give an indication of how long it will keep safe for eating.

Nutrient requirements

Nutrients are substances that are essential for life. They are needed in order for animals to live, grow and reproduce. There are five main categories of nutrient.

Protein

Proteins are workhorses of the body and perform many different, complex functions in a body's cells. Amongst other things they help repair and replace the cells that make up muscle, tissue, blood and bone.

Proteins are made from different combinations of chemicals called amino acids. Animals' bodies can make many amino acids but not all of them. The amino acids that cannot be made must be obtained from food instead. Different species have different requirements – essential amino acids for a cat may not be essential for, say, a dog. The dietary requirements of a cat are therefore different to those of a dog.

Essential amino acids can be obtained from both plant and animal sources – fish, meat, dairy, pulses and cereals.

Proteins can also be used by the body as a source of energy if other sources – e.g. carbohydrates and fat – have run out. Excess protein is not stored in the body, however, and is excreted from the body in urine.

Fats

A group of molecules known as fatty acids consist of long chains of hydrogen and carbon atoms, arranged in different ways. Fats are made up up from different arrangements of fatty acids.

Fats are classified as **saturated** or

unsaturated, according to the chemical structure of the fatty acids that they are made from. Saturated fats are solid at room temperature and usually found in meat and dairy products. Unsaturated fats are liquid at room temperature and are usually found in vegetable products and fish.

Fats are a concentrated form of energy and can be stored under the skin. Fats are also essential to the absorption of vitamins A, D, E and K. Different animals need particular fats and some can only be obtained from their diet.

Fats provide insulation for animals and protects their internal organs from external impact. Certain types of fats are also important elements within cell membranes.

Carbohydrates

Carbohydrates are molecules made up of carbon, hydrogen and oxygen atoms. They are an important source of energy for animals.

There are many different forms of carbohydrate. Some have very simple chemical structures, such as sugars. Simple sugars are absorbed quickly and easily by the body after eating.

Other carbohydrates have far more complex chemical structures, such as starch and cellulose. Starch is found in lots of foodstuff, such as rice, cereals, grains and bread. It takes longer for the body to break it down during digestion because it is a complex carbohydrate.

Cellulose is another complex carbohydrate. It makes up the cell walls in plants. It is a structure that gives vegetables their 'crunch' but it cannot be digested by humans or most animals. However some animals, such as cows, sheep and goats, have special digestion processes that can break cellulose down. For other animals cellulose is still useful because it acts a source of dietary fibre – something which aids the digestion process.

Minerals, vitamins and trace elements

Animals' bodies need to eat protein, fats and carbohydrates in relatively large amounts.

However they also need much smaller amounts of a large range of other substances. These can be categorised as vitamins or minerals.

Minerals are chemical elements that the body needs. For instance, bones in the body are made from the chemical element calcium. Calcium is, therefore a an important mineral that can only be obtained from food. Any mineral that is needed in absolutely tiny amounts is called a trace element. Most minerals needed by animals are trace elements - only a few minerals are needed in larger amounts.

'Vitamin' is a broad name for other nutrients needed by the body in small amounts. They are each made from different chemicals, perform different functions and are given special names. For instance, vitamin A is important for reproduction, and keeping skin, fur and coats in good condition.

Vitamins and minerals are not sources of energy but can help the body release energy from other sources.

Consuming too much of any mineral, and some vitamins, can cause health problems. These amounts will differ from species to species.

Dietary requirements

Animals' bodies rely on obtaining nutrients in the correct amounts in order to live healthy lives and prevent malnutrition or obesity. Different animal species require different amounts of each nutrient and so a diet that is suitable for one species is unlikely to be suitable for another. For instance, cats need much larger amounts of protein than dogs. Even within the same species, animals' nutritional needs can be different.

Beyond species, there are a number of factors that determine animal dietary requirements.

Size and weight

Larger animals would normally have higher energy needs and require more food in a typical day. For instance it is natural for a large dog to eat more than a small dog.

However, an animal that is overweight or obese will require a diet that is lower in energy than a healthy animal, so that it can lose weight.

Age

Younger animals often need more energy than adults to help with growth and because they are very active. Older animals are normally less active and need less energy in their diet.

Activity levels

The more active an animal is, the more energy it will need. This may be down to natural differences - for instance, some breeds of dog are just more active than others. But it can also be down to the kind of life they lead - for instance a 'house cat' will walk much less than a stray cat.

Working animals require more energy than non-working animals.

Parturition

Parturition means giving birth. Animals that are pregnant, or are feeding their young, have very specific nutritional needs that are different to a typical adult of their species. Their energy needs are higher.

Number and frequency of feeds

The number of feeds, and how often depend on a number of things including:

- nutritional requirements
- the number of animals feeding at the same time

- how well the feed keeps - i.e. whether food can be left out or not
- animals' feeding behaviour - for instance, whether they will overeat if food is made available for a longer period of time
- schedule - feeding may need to fit around other activities.

Correct storage

As has been discussed, different types of food keep for different lengths of time. Food must be stored in an appropriate way so that it keeps as expected. This might mean, for instance, keeping dried food sealed and away from water, as it is likely to spoil if it becomes wet, and keeping fresh food refrigerated.

Jargon Buster

longevity how long something will keep for

sugars simple carbohydrates

starch a complex carbohydrate

cellulose a complex carbohydrate found in plant material that most animals cannot digest

complex carbohydrate a carbohydrate with a more complicated molecular structure

trace element minerals that are essential for life but required in very small amounts

malnutrition a health condition due to a diet insufficient in essential nutrients

parturition birth

amino acid chemicals that make up proteins

Quiz Questions

1 a) Why might a farmer choose to feed her cows with haylage? b) What time of year is she most likely to do so?

2 Why is protein particularly important for an animal recovering from an injury?

3 What nutritional requirements might a large, young animal have compared to a small fully-grown adult animal of the same species?

1.2 Prepare equipment to feed and water animals

In this topic you will learn about selecting and preparing feeding and watering equipment:

* utensils, bowls, troughs, automatic feeders, hay nets, buckets, automatic water containers and bottles

You will learn to take into account:

* species

* design

* construction materials

* cleaning requirements

* hygiene and disinfection

* storage

Selecting and preparing equipment to feed and water animals

Once the type, quantity and frequency of food has been chosen, you need to consider how that food will be delivered to animals. There are a range of options depending on species and lifestyle.

Utensils, bowls and buckets

For companion animals a wide variety of small bowls, dishes and utensils are available for food and water.

Similarly, for livestock, the simplest container in which to provide food or water is a plastic or metal bucket.

Troughs

For livestock, where the numbers of animals feeding at the same time are much greater, feeding troughs are a good way to distribute food. The troughs need to be large enough to accommodate all animals feeding at the same time.

Automatic feeders

Automatic feeding equipment uses technology to release food to animals at certain times of day, as specified by the user. More sophisticated equipment can also vary the amount of food released.

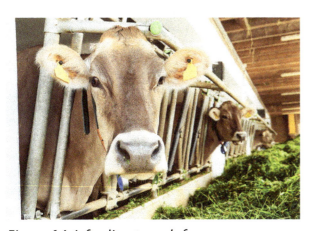

Figure 14 A feeding trough for cows

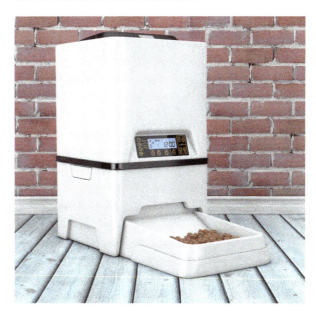

Figure 15 An automatic food dispenser

43

This is useful for livestock because it cuts down on the amount of time that needs to be spent each day feeding animals - instead the automatic feeders can be filled every few days. For companion animals, automatic feeders allow owners to leave them for a longer period of time.

By feeding smaller amounts more frequently, automatic feeders also help to keep food free from contamination.

Automatic water containers and bottles

Water is particularly prone to contamination if left in bowls or troughs and dirty water can cause serious ill health. Just like automatic feeders, automatic water containers can provide fresh water at regular intervals. Water bottles also keep water free from contamination and supply water 'on-demand' whenever the animal wants it.

Hay nets

Hay nets are used to slow down eating times for animals such as horses. The smaller the holes in the net, the longer it takes the animal to pull out the hay. Because grazing animals evolved to eat small amounts of food

frequently, hay nets can be seen as a more natural way to feed such animals.

Considerations to take into account

Deciding which equipment to choose will depend on the following.

Species requirements

The needs of the animal are the most important thing to consider when choosing the most suitable feeding equipment. You should think about the following:

- Animal diets: as we have seen animals can be fed different kinds of food. This has an impact on the equipment used to deliver it.

- The size of the animal: particularly for young animals, will they be able to reach the food and water?

- The number of animals feeding at one time: will there be space for all of them?

- The amount of food and water that will served at feeding time: will the container be big enough?

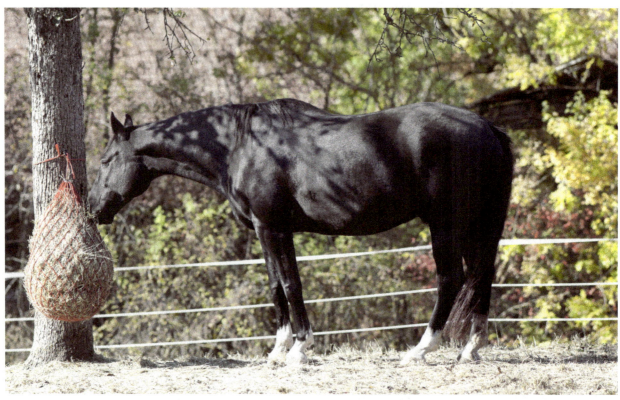

Figure 16 A horse feeding from a hay net

44

- Special dietary needs: do some animals need feeding separately? Are some animals obese?

- Natural feeding behaviour: should animals be fed smaller portions over the day? Will they simply eat everything that is there? Are they agressive with each other at mealtimes? Are there submissive animals that will not get a fair share of food?

Design

Clever designs will keep food and water in the best possible condition for as long as possible. They will also minimise spillage and waste. Food waste attracts vermin such as rats who also bring disease.

In the wild, most animals spend much of their time finding food. It can lead to boredom when food is simply provided for them. For some species it might be appropriate to consider feeding equipment that is designed to occupy them for longer.

The design should ensure that food and water is always available, i.e that blockages do not occur.

Construction materials

There is often a choice between metal and plastic. Metal is more expensive but more robust. This means that it will last longer but also protect food from unwanted visitors such as rats. It is also heavier, which can prevent the feeding equipment from being knocked over. However, some metals will corrode when exposed to the elements.

Cleaning requirements, hygiene and disinfection

Out-of-date food is a health hazard, so feeding equipment has to be emptied and cleaned regularly. Equipment should be easy to take apart for washing, cleaning and drying of all components. Any equipment that is hard to clean is a breeding ground for bacteria and other microorganisms.

Storage

Even food with a long shelf-life will deteriorate quickly in the wrong conditions. Equipment for storing food should be air-tight, free from moisture and inaccesible to vermin.

Jargon Buster

submissive when animals give way to other animals to avoid conflict

vermin carriers of disease - typically refers to wild mice and rats

corrode the deterioration of a material through a chemical reaction - for example, rust

Quiz Questions

1 List the benefits of using an automatic feeder.

2 Name three items of feeding equipment.

3 Describe two considerations to bear in mind when selecting suitable feeding equipment.

LO2 Feed and monitor animals

2.1 Plan diets for animals

In this topic you will learn about

- planning diets for animals for maintenance and according to life stage and specific nutritional needs

- differences in diet from normal adult diet for: pregnant animals, lactating animals, geriatric animals, ill/injured animals, animals in recovery from illness/operation, young animals, change in activity/purpose/use of animal (working/non-working, competition).

Planning diets for maintenance and according to life stage and nutritional needs

We have seen that different animal species require different quantities of nutrients such as protein, fat and carbohydrate, in order to maintain a healthy lifestyle. These quantities are based on an average, healthy adult animal from the species. However, individual animals may have slightly different requirements if they are not 'average healthy adults'. These differences may be down to lifestyle, life stage (i.e. age), or other specific nutritional needs.

Some of the most important factors are considered below. Whilst the general trends are discussed, you **must** carefully research and understand the nutritional requirements of your chosen species at each life stage **as there may be differences from the general cases stated here.**

Pregnant animals

The demands of pregnancy means that more energy is required by pregnant animals and new mothers. The exact details depend on species however. For instance, pregnant dogs gain most of their weight in the final part of pregnancy, and this is when they need the greatest additional energy. In the early stage of pregancy their additional energy needs can be quite small. In contrast, cats require increasing amounts of energy in the very early stages of pregancy. It is to be noted however that, despite higher energy needs, overfeeding pregnant animals can prove to be

dangerous to the mother and her offspring.

It is usual to provide smaller portions of food more frequently for pregnant animals, to aid digestion. This is because there is not as much room as normal for digestive organs at the end of the pregnancy, so mothers will get full very quickly. For the same reason, the digestibility of food is important at the later stages of pregnancy.

Aside from energy, higher proportions of other nutrients may be important, such as protein and calcium. Commercially available food labelled as 'complete' for pregnancy contains the correct proportions of all necessary nutrients for that particular species.

Lactating animals

Lactating means producing milk, and it can require even more nutritional energy than pregnancy itself. For instance dogs may need 2-4 times more energy when lactating than normal. With such high energy needs it may be necessary to ensure food is available to eat at all times.

All animals should have easy access to fresh drinking water at all times. Lactating animals will become dehydrated more quickly and will consume more water - so water levels should be checked even more regularly.

Geriatric animals

Geriatric means 'old'. Older animals tend to become less active, which means that they need less energy. If they consume the same amount of energy as when they were younger, they are likely to put on weight, which is a serious health risk. Food for older animals tends to have fewer carbohydrates and contain less energy.

Older animals may find it harder to digest food as they get older, so diets with higher fibre may be appropriate, along with greater quantities of water. If older animals are not drinking enough then more moisture may need to be provided in their food.

Specialised feeds are available, specifically formulated for older animals.

Animals in recovery from illness, operation or injury

Sick animals need nutrients in order to get better. They may, however, have lost their appetite, so their food needs to be attractive to eat (palatable) and easily digestible. This tends to mean an increased proportion of fat and a decreased proportion of carbohydrates. However, as sick animals will not be active, their overall energy requirement may be decreased.

Animals with wounds need protein to help repair tissue. Dehydration is a serious concern for sick animals and needs to be carefully monitored.

Juvenile animals

Juvenile means 'young'. Juvenile animals are not just maintaining their body, they are growing rapidly and need more energy to fuel this growth. This means proportionally more carbohydrate and fat than for adults. They also need proportionally more protein for building new tissue. They will often need more minerals and vitamins than adults as well.

So, by percentage of the weight of the food, juveniles tend to need more of everything!

However they also have relatively small stomachs and can't eat much food in one go. So they need to be fed small portions at regular intervals.

As with other life stages, feeds formulated for common species of juvenile animals are available.

Change in activity, purpose and use of animal

A typical adult's energy requirement is based on a typical amount of daily activity, as appropriate for that species. So, for a companion animal like a dog, this would be based on one or two bouts of exercise a day. A working dog however would be far more active than this and burn off more energy in a working day - and therefore their nutritonal needs would include a greater percentage of carbohydrates than a typical dog. Similarly, a racehorse has far higher energy needs than a normal horse.

However, a working dog or racehorse that had retired would no longer use up so much energy and would need fewer carbohydrates than before. In this way, the nutritional demands of animals will change as their activity or purpose changes over time, and this means their diet also has to change. The exact details depend, of course, on the species and the activity.

Jargon Buster

lactating the process of making milk for young to feed on - only mammals lactate

geriatric another term for old

juvenile another term for young

palatable the attractiveness of food

Quiz Questions

1 Explain why planning a diet for a pregnant cow would require special consideration.

2 Why do lactating animals require special diets?

3 A recently retired greyhound has been adopted by a young couple. Discuss the advice you would give to help plan meals..

2.2 Provide food and water to animals

In this topic you will learn about the following aspects of providing food and water to animals:

- **Feeding times**

- **Preparation of animal ration/meal**

- **Food for training/treats, enrichment**

- **Supplements and other dietary essentials (cuttlefish, grit)**

- **Delivery of feed to animals**

- **Feeding individuals and groups**

- **Checking animals are eating**

- **Cleaning feeding utensils and equipment**

- **Storage of feeding utensils and equipment**

- **Checking water availability**

- **Providing fresh water and cleaning watering equipment**

- **Correct monitoring and disposal of waste feed (incorporating good practice of disposal methods)**

Food and water is normally provided to animals as part of a feeding plan. When designing a feeding plan, all aspects of feeding must be considered, not just the nutritional aspects. The common aspects are discussed below. All of them need to be considered in relation to your chosen species.

Feeding times

Choosing when and how often to feed animals is an important consideration and is related to the nutritional needs, life stages and number of animals, as well as consideration of the animal's natural feeding habits in the wild. Foraging animals, for instance, have evolved to eat fairly continuously - not just one meal a day. The practicalities of actually delivering food will of course also have a big impact.

Food may need delivering at certain times of the day, or more frequently than just once. It is common for feeding times to stay roughly the same each day for animals that benefit

from a routine.

Preparation of animal meals

When preparing food for animals there are a number of things to consider.

Following the plan

Food needs to be prepared exactly as per the feeding plan. Any special dietary requirements can be catered for and any supplements added at this point.

Hazards to human health

There are potential hazards to human health, including:

Handling heavy or dangerous equipment and utensils. Health and safety measures should be in place to minimise risks when using or moving potentially dangerous or heavy equipment. This might include things like:

- storing heavy items close to where they are used

- understanding the correct posture for carrying or operating machines

- ensuring more than one person is available to help with heavy items

- suitable rules around using knives and other sharp equipment and machines

Risk of infection. People working with food must follow stringent hygiene practices for their own health (as well as the animals'). For instance, contamination from raw meat is a serious health risk and so meat hygiene practices requires raw and cooked food to be kept completely separate, with different implements and surfaces used for each. Hands should be thoroughly washed after handling any raw meat.

Disposal of wasted food must also be done safely so as not to endanger humans or animals that may come into contact with it.

There may be other hazards in the food preparation area, such as the generation of dust from food products and repetitive motions that can cause muscle or skeletal injuries.

There is always a risk of infectious diseases being passed between animals and humans and vice versa. A full risk assessment must be performed to identify all potential hazards and full health and safety training is required for all staff. Personal Protective Equipment (PPE) may need to be worn.

Hazards to animal health

The food hygiene practices described above are also in place to protect the animals' health. Contamination of food stuff is a constant threat, so all food must be assessed for:

- Shelf life - is the food too old to eat? Is meat safe to eat? Meat should always be carefully assessed regardless of the stated shelf life.

- Contamination - has the food been attacked by vermin such as rats? Have any substances accidentally spoiled the food? (Even a substance such as water can spoil dried food.) It is assumed that vermin will

always be present wherever food is stored and so measures should be in place to control potential pests.

Anyone cooking must know how to prepare and cook food safely. This is particularly true for:

- Meat - is it cooked thoroughly, in line with the dietary requirements of the species? Raw meat should always be prepared completely separately from other food, using completely separate cooking implements.

- Frozen food - there are particular ways in which frozen food can and cannot be cooked.

All equipment and surfaces used for food preparation must be kept clean and hygienic.

Waste

Food preparation should be planned carefully and efficiently so that quantities are correct and any waste is minimised.

Food for training, treats, enrichment

Food can be used as a reward for animal behaviour. It can be used to motivate an animal to learn, and therefore allows animals to be trained. It works through positive reinforcement - the animal learns that if they repeat a certain behaviour there will be a reward at the end. Food is partcularly useful for this because there is such a strong instinct to eat or to find food.

Given that food is supplied every day regardless of behaviour, it is normal to use special treats for training. This would consist of food that the animal places a high value on, and is not normally available. For instance, a cat that is normally fed dry food will respond very positively to a little cooked fresh meat. Many different treats are commercially available which are designed to be highly attractive to the species in question. That attraction is due to a high number of calories and a higher level of fat content. As a result treats should be given only occasionally.

In the wild, animals spend a great deal of time

49

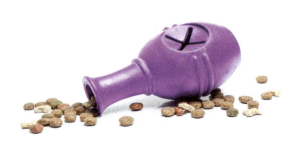

Figure 17 Food puzzle toy for a dog

finding and eating food. The process of doing so is often very mentally stimulating for them. Animals in captivity, however, are provided with food and can become bored as a result. This can lead to more serious behavioural issues. Mealtimes can be made more interesting and mentally enriching through the thoughtful delivery of food. Delivering food in a way that can stimulate an animal will help prevent boredom and lengthen meal times, which may prevent over-eating.

For instance, food can be scattered around the environment so that animals have to find it, rather than having it all placed in one feeding bowl. It can also be hidden, which will encourage foraging behaviour. Food can also be supplied in dispensing toys, where an animal has to interact with the toy in order to eat. This makes feeding time exciting and interesting.

There are also puzzle feeders available, where the animal is rewarded with food once they have figured out how the feeder works. However, food must not be so well hidden that it stops the animal from eating and fresh water does need to easily available at all times.

Supplements and other dietary essentials

Supplements refers to additional ingredients added to, or in addition, to normal feeding. Nutritional supplements may be required if the normal feed does not contain all of the necessary nutrients for that animal. For instance, an animal may have a health condition that requires them to consume

additional vitamins. Alternatively, cattle that are primarily fed on grass may need supplementary food in winter, depending on the purpose of the animal.

For livestock animals, decisions regarding supplements are also affected by the chosen method of farming. For instance certain supplements may be needed for animals that are intensively farmed compared to those who are not.

For a companion animal, supplements are unecessary if they are being fed a 'complete' diet that matches their age, lifestyle and activity level.

It is important to note that some vitamins and all minerals are stored in the body. Consuming too much of any of them can have serious health consequences and so great care must be taken when considering adding any supplements to an animal's diet.

Cuttlefish

A cuttlefish or cuttlebone is made from the shell of an animal called a cuttlefish and is used for birds, and some other animals such as turtles, as source of dietary calcium and othe minerals. The act of eating it also helps birds to maintain a healthy beak.

Grit

Some animals require supplements not for nutrition but to help them to digest food. For instance, birds do not have teeth to break up their food and need to use grit or cuttlefish to help them do so. The mechanical action of food grinding against grit or cuttlefish helps to break it down into smaller pieces. Grit is insoluble, which means it does not dissolve and cannot be digested.

Whilst some birds in the wild naturally consume grit when foraging for food, there is some debate over whether grit is necessary for birds in captivity given that their food is often processed in some way.

Delivery of feed to animals

You must consider how food will be delivered to animals. If there are multiple animals then provisions must be in place to ensure all animal have equal access. Consideration must be given to animals who have special requirements or conditions that might make feeding difficult. If there is unlikely to be enough room around one feeding station then multiple stations must be included.

Food can be delivered to animals in different ways and the plan must cover this. When delivering food there is an opportunity to think of creative enrichment activities in which an animal could be stimulated at the same time, as discussed earlier.

Feeding individuals and groups

Feeding animals individually means that you can be sure that the correct portion is fed at the correct time. For livestock animals it is not practical to feed them individually and certain measures need to be in place to ensure all animals receive food as outlined in a feeding plan.

The most important point is that all animals must be able to access the feeding station. This means considering the accessibility of the feeding equipment - for instance, is it too high for young animals? - and whether each animal has enough room. There may be a 'pecking order' when groups of animals eat together, in which case you need to be sure enough food is available for the last animal to eat. If any animal is not receiving its fair share then feeding may need to split into smaller groups which take place at different times or separate locations. If one animal is dominating at feed time, or young animals are being bullied, then they may need feeding separately.

If animals within a group have very different nutrional needs then it is unlikely that one feed will be sufficient for all of them; again feeding should be split into groups, with each group made up of animals with similar nutritional needs.

Checking animals are eating

Designing and delivering a perfect feeding routine is of little use if animals are not eating in the way that was envisaged. It is very important therefore that animals' feeding habits are monitored:

- The amount of food eaten. This might be a visual inspection and might include weighing food quantities before and after.

- The type of food eaten. If there is a choice of several different foods, are animals selectively eating some but not others? If so this will lead to an unbalanced diet.

- Has there been any change in feeding patterns or behaviour? Any such changes can be an indicator of a health problem or a behavioural condition.

Checking the consumption of water is also very important, particularly as weather changes over the course of a year. Sometimes a change in eating patterns is caused by limited access to water.

Consideration needs to be made as to how regularly to check all of this and to time the checks consistently. Only by being consistent can you pick up on genuine changes in behaviour rather than variances caused by, for example, the time of the day.

As a result of these checks it may be that the feeding routine needs to be changed.

Cleaning feeding utensils and equipment

Feeding equipment and utsensils can quickly become dirty. This might be due to the presence of old food or it might be due to animals contaminating equipment with droppings, fur, soil etc. All of these are a potential source of harmful microorganisms and so all equipment used to prepare food and feed animals needs to be kept clean. It may not be practical to clean every piece of equipment before and after every feed. However a cleaning routine should be established so that all pieces of equipment are cleaned frequently and to make sure that none are missed.

Storage of feeding utensils and equipment

Any excess food needs to be removed from all utensils and equipment, which should then be thoroughly cleaned, washed and dried. Equipment should be stored in dry

51

locations away from vermin or other sources of contamination.

Any stored food should be labelled clearly.

Providing and checking fresh water availability and cleaning watering equipment

Water is essential for animals, so fresh, clean water must be made available for all animals at all times. Contaminated water poses a risk to health so the water container itself, and any other equipment used to provide water, must be kept clean and hygienic at all times. Animals are prone to contaminate water themselves, so it must be checked for cleanliness as well as availablility at regular intervals.

Correct monitoring and disposal of waste feed

Waste animal feed must be disposed of safely so that it doesn't pose a threat to human or animal health. Any waste with potential for transmission of disease needs to be stored in suitable containers. Particular care must be taken for food containing animal by-products as their disposal is heavily regulated to ensure that such products do not end back up in the animal or human food chain.

Plant-based waste material can be suitable for composting and containers that are no longer needed should be considered for recycling.

Different types of food waste need to be clearly labelled, which could be done using colour-coded bins.

Jargon Buster
contamination spreading germs from one item or surface to another

Quiz Questions

1 Describe how feeding times could help enrich an animal's experience.

2 List three considerations to take into account when preparing animals' food.

3 Describe two possible hazards to health posed by animal food.

2.3 The importance of monitoring, recording and reporting on food and water intake

In this topic you will learn:

- **How to monitor animals' food and water intake - food and water intake and timescales, intake of supplements (vitamins, minerals, oils).**

- **How to record animals' food and water intake - type of information to be recorded (amount given and left and feeding behaviour), frequency of records, display or storage of records**

- **About reporting appropriately on any problems which are likely to occur if an inadequate or inappropriate diet has been provided.**

- **About symptoms of inadequate or inappropriate nutrition: stress, hair/fur/feather loss, obesity, disease or illness, low immunity, malnutrition, death, problems with breeding or pregnancy, change in temperament, swimming abnormalities, pica/coprophagia.**

Once a feeding plan is in place and is being delivered it must be monitored and recorded. This is to ensure that the plan is effective. Even effective plans will need to change over time, as animals' bodies and behaviour change. Monitoring and recording will inform if and when a plan has to change. It also allows potential health problems to be picked up, possibly before any other symptoms are present.

Sometimes monitoring may find issues that only occur occasionally or that are not specified in the feeding plan. For instance:

- Poor preparation - food that is not easy to physically eat for some reason, e.g. it has not been peeled or needs to be in smaller chunks.

- Quality issues - food that has spoiled in some way between storage, preparation and delivery.

- Delivery issues - sometimes the way in which food is delivered can affect an animal's feeding behaviour, for instance delivering the food in a different location. Alternatively a piece of delivery equipment may have broken which stops animals eating as normal.

Health and behavioural reasons for a change in appetite will be discussed shortly.

How to monitor and record animals' food and water intake

Food and water intake and timescales

Anyone directly involved in caring for an animal is in a good position to monitor their feeding behaviour, and any changes to that behaviour. Questions to consider include:

- how much food was eaten?

- how much water was drunk?

- were there any perceived changes in appetite?

- was there any unusual behaviour when eating?

- were there any changes in food/water consumption that were unusual for that animal?

- were there any unusual substances present e.g. blood or vomit?

Such monitoring would normally take place during and after feeding time. Consideration should be made for typical behaviour in the species. For instance, if a particular species tends to eat their food over the course of a day then monitoring their intake straight after feeding is unlikely to pick up on any changes in behaviour.

It is also important to ensure that intake is monitored before food and water implements are emptied and cleaned.

Intake of supplements

When animals are given additional supplements as part of their feeding plan, such as vitamins, minerals and oils, their consumption needs to be monitored in much the same way as for food and water.

Information to be recorded

Recording food and water intake allows you to keep track of feeding behaviour over time. It is very important as it provides detailed and accurate information that relates to the specific animals being cared for. It is also very useful when more than one person cares for an animal, as it provides a full picture of feeding behaviour which one person may miss. Objectively measured data, such as quantities of food, provide hard evidence that can indicate any potential health or behavioural conditions. More subjective behavioural observations are also important.

Data that is normally recorded includes:

- The quantity of food provided, and left, (normally by mass i.e. grams or kilograms).

- If there was anything different to normal about the delivered food then that should be recorded too.

- How much of the food was eaten. An agreed scale can be used as long as it is consistently applied - for instance a 0-3 rating could be used where '0' means 'did not eat anything' and '3' means 'ate all the food provided'.

- Feeding behaviour. Are animals anticipating feeding time? Are they eating food enthusiastically or do they appear disinterested? Are there changes in their normal behaviour when being fed? When there are choices of food, are some elements left until last or not eaten at all?

- The amount of water given and amount left. As water should always be available, some water should always remain at each observation.

Another way to track the impact of diet is to record the appearance of faecal matter. The consistency of faeces can indicate if an animal is getting enough water or is constipated. A more technical analysis can indicate if certain nutrients are not being digested by the animal, which may then require dietary changes. Changes in faeces can indicate dietary, health or behavioural issues (such as stress).

Frequency of records

Recording would normally take place at least once per feeding session. As ever, there may be exceptions specific to a particular species.

Display or storage of records

Records may be paper-based, electronic or both. In all cases records should be easily accessible for all relevant staff, and any external parties who may require access (such as a vet). They should be easy for third parties to interpret and easily identifiable with each animal.

For paper-based records meaures should be taken to ensure they cannot be damaged or lost - for instance record cards by an animal's cage must be protected from rain and from the animal itself. Duplicates should be made just in case. Similarly, for electronic storage there must be a system in place in the event of a catastrophic failure of equipment. In practice this normally means backing up data on a daily basis.

Reporting appropriately on any problems if an inadequate or inappropriate diet has been provided.

Recording data is of no use without knowing what to do with the information. A system should be in place so that everyone knows what to do with the findings.

Sometimes the monitoring and recording will discover serious issues that need addressing immediately. For instance, an animal might be observed to be seriously dehydrated. Simply providing more water might not be a solution because the issue might be a more general health problem. As dehydration can quickly cause serious health problems, such an issue needs to be raised straightaway with a senior member of staff. Such conditions or behaviour will be defined as 'top priority', requiring immediate intervention and reporting.

Reporting other observations will depend on the seriousness of their impact over a certain timeframe. All records would normally be reviewed at regular intervals and some observations can be addressed then. For instance if an animal has left a small amount of food on one day then that might not be an immediate cause for concern. If it happens consistently over a week then a review of the records might decide to implement gradual changes to that animal's feed. Alternatively, if an animal begins to leave more and more food each day then that might require more rapid action and might need reporting sooner.

Whilst each organisation will define how best to report on any signs of an inadequate or inappropriate diet, if you have any concerns about the importance of an observation then you should report it to a senior member of staff as soon as you can.

Symptoms of inadequate or inappropriate nutrition

Stress

A number of different factors can cause stress in animals, including a poor diet, or restrictions to natural feeding behaviour.

The symptoms of stress include:

- pacing up and down or round and round, rocking back and forth
- repeated unusual or excessive vocalisations
- cowering
- repeated biting or tongue movements
- excessive grooming
- trying to escape
- unusually timid or trembling
- loss of appetite.

Other sources of stress, aside from nutrition, should also be considered for any animals

displaying symptoms.

Hair/fur/feather loss

Loss of hair, fur or feathers can be due to nutritional deficiencies in the diet. Nutrients that contribute to healthy skin and coat include:

- high-quality protein
- essential fatty acids
- vitamin E
- vitamin A
- vitamin B6
- zinc
- copper

(These nutrients contribute to many other aspects of a healthy lifestyle too!)

Another cause of hair, fur or feather loss is excessive grooming due to stress. Such stress may be due to a poor diet or may be due to some other circumstances.

Problems with hair, fur or feathers can also be due to parasites such as ticks and lice.

Obesity

Animals that are consistently consuming more energy than they need will gain weight. This may be seen visually or through measurement i.e. weighing. Obesity is a serious condition that carries many health risks for an animal and must be addressed.

Malnutrition, disease and illness

Malnutrition is a general condition caused by nutrient deficiency or over-consumption of nutrients. This in turn can result in any number of diseases, illnesses or conditions.

Correct quantities of nutrients differ between species. There are too many to list here, but some common nutrients, and symptoms of inadequate provision, are:

- Proteins - essential for repair of tissue and almost all bodily processes, lack of protein can lead to impaired vision and tooth decay.
- Vitamin A - a lack of vitamin A leads

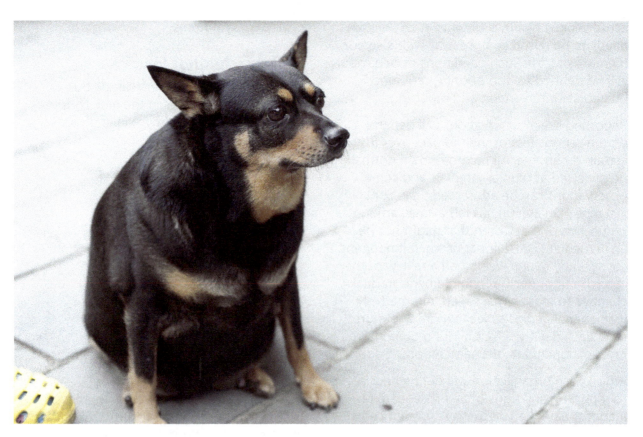

Figure 18 This dog's health is at risk because it is obsese

to night blindness, problems with reproduction, bad condition of hair and skin.

- Vitamin D - inadequate amounts lead to weak and curved bones, growth problems, weak legs.

- Vitamin B12 - lack of B12 leads to growth problems, lack of oxygen in the blood (anaemia), loss of appetite.

- Calcium - as the skeleton is constructed using calcium, deficiencies lead to problems with the bones and teeth.

- Potassium - inadequate amounts can lead to paralysis, loss of muscle mass, urinating frequently, thirst.

- Zinc - a lack of zinc can lead to lesions, poor skin condition and a dull coat.

Disease and illness can also be caused by over-consumption of some nutrients. For instance, obesity is caused by eating too much fat and/or carbohydrates. Over-consumption of certain vitamins - those which are fat-soluble and are stored in the body - can also lead to health problems.

Low immunity

The immune system works to protect an animal's body from disease caused by pathogens, such as viruses and bacteria. It is made up of a complex combination of chemical processes in the body. These processes rely on a full range of nutrients from a balanced diet. Malnutrition (including over-consumption) has an overall negative effect on the immune system. This means that, quite apart from the direct health impacts, animals with poor diets are also more likely to get ill from a wide range of transmitted diseases.

Problems with breeding or pregnancy

As we have already seen, pregnant animals have very specific nutritional requirements. These requirements are to ensure the health of the offspring and of the mother. However, even before becoming pregnant, breeding animals have particular nutritional needs that will make pregnancy more likely.

Malnourished animals do not have sufficient quantities of important nutrients, such as protein, to fully support the initial development of a foetus or the growth of an embryo later on. It also impacts on how many embryos a mother can support. Malnourishment is a major contributor to birth defects, miscarriage and problems with lactating/nursing offspring.

Change in temperament

Diet can impact on temperament and behaviour. For instance carboydrates can be in complex forms (starch, cellulose) or simple forms (sugars). In mammals, just as in humans, simple carbohydrates are quickly broken down by the body and absorbed into the bloodstream. Too many simple carbohydrates lead to rapid increases and decreases in blood sugar levels, which itself can cause erratic mood swings and boosts or crashes in energy.

Other nutrients may also affect temperament. For instance there are some studies that make a connection between a high-protein diet in dogs and higher levels of aggression.

If there are changes to an animal's temperament then careful analysis of any dietary changes should be made, in case there is a link between the two.

Swimming abnormalities

Swim bladder disorders are fairly common in fish. The swim bladder is an organ that allows a fish to keep a netutral buoyancy, which stops them from sinking to the bottom or floating to the top of the water. The fish can allow air in and out of the bladder as it is needed. Any problem with the swim bladder can affect the ability of a fish to swim correctly, which can include:

- swimming on one side
- swimming with the head higher than the tail or vice versa
- floating at the top or sinking to the bottom
- swimming upside down.

Food delivered as flakes that float on the surface of the water can cause the condition if fish take in too much air when they eat. Alternatively some dry food can expand in water and cause the fish's stomach to bloat, which can then press on the swim bladder.

Pica and coprophagia

Pica is a condition whereby animals eat non-food items that have no nutritional value, such as stones or soil. Coprophagia is the name given to eating excrement or faeces. Whilst coprophagia is natural for some animals (such as rabbits), in general both pica and coprophagia are potentially dangerous because of the parasites present in faeces and the physical damage that foreign objects can do to the digestive system.

Each condition can be caused by malnutrition - i.e. if a diet is deficient in some way then an animals may attempt to supplement their food with whatever they find.

Other causes of both conditions include underlying health issues or behavioural problems. (Also see Unit 201 section 3.2).

Death

In extreme cases a poor diet can ultimately lead to death.

Jargon Buster

pathogen an organism that causes disease

pica eating non-food objects

coprophagia eating faeces

faeces poo

vocalisation noises made with the mouth

Quiz Questions

1 List three symptoms that might indicate stress.

2 Name three things that you would expect to be monitored in a typical feeding plan.

3 What are the dangers for an animal displaying pica?

4 Why might a fish swimming on one side be a sign of an inappropriate diet?

5 What should you do if you suspect an animal is dehydrated?

LO3 Clean and prepare animal accommodation

3.1 Types of animal housing

In this topic you will learn about the construction and design of different animal housing:

- Materials - wood, glass, metal and plastic.

- Structure and design - moveable and immoveable, location, weight, sufficient space, strength, safety, security and access, ease of cleaning, weatherproofing and drainage, waste disposal, location of services, purpose of accommodation, suitability for the animals and cost.

- Environmental factors - wind direction, humidity, ventilation, temperature and light, neighbours and pollution.

- Welfare factors - species-specific requirements, conforms to the five welfare needs .

- Fixtures and fittings (bedding and substrate, hides, beds or boxes, ladders, ramps and levels, enrichment items, lighting and heating, natural furnishings)

Construction and design of different animal housing types

Animal accommodation is the environment in which an animal lives. It is often made up of a primary and secondary enclosure. The primary enclosure is the immediate space which the animal has access to and the secondary enclosure is the space in which the primary enclosure is placed. Both primary and secondary enclosures need to be designed and constructed with a number of factors in mind, to provide animals with a safe, clean, hygienic and stress-free environment.

Examples of animal accommodation include:

- cages
- indoor pens
- stalls
- outdoor runs
- kennels
- aviaries
- hutches
- vivariums/terrariums.

Materials

The first thing to consider is what material, or mix of materials, to construct accommodation from. The properties of the most common materials are described below.

Wood

Advantages

- Cheap.
- Easy to work with.
- Wide variety of structures can be built from it.
- As a natural material, wooden structures look attractive and can blend in if attempting to create a natural-looking environment.

Disadvantages

- Some animals will enjoy gnawing or scratching wooden structures. This may be enjoyable for the animal but means the structure can be destroyed over time.
- Not very durable - will need to be treated to protect from the environment e.g. rain.

- Wood can be sharp and splinters can cause injuries.

- Not easy to clean or disinfect, so germs can easily multiply on surfaces.

- There is always a risk of fire with wooden structures.

Glass

Advantages

- Cheap.

- Durable - can withstand the elements.

- Escape-proof.

- Easy to clean and disinfect.

- Provides natural light whilst retaining heat.

- Smooth surfaces means animals are unlikely to cut themselves.

- Modern glass is shatter-proof in case of an accident.

Disadvantages

- Harder to work into non-standard shapes.

- Air-tight so ventilation must be provided.

- Spaces can heat up to dangerous levels in direct sunlight or hot days.

- Because it is transparent animals can sometimes injure themselves if they don't realise it is there.

Metal

There are different types of metal, such as aluminium and stainless steel, that have different properties but some common advantages and disadvantages are:

Advantages

- Suitable metals are durable against the elements and animals.

- Easy to clean and disinfect.

- Smooth surfaces means animals are unlikely to cut themselves.

- Escape-proof.

- Some metals are relatively inexpensive.

Disadvantages

- Some metals are relatively expensive.

- Harder to cut and shape to size than wood.

- Some metals are heavy.

- Metals block all light.

Plastic

As with metal, there are many different types of plastic that each have slightly different properties. Common plastic used for animal housing include fibreglass and PVC.

Advantages

- Cheap.

- Durable against the elements.

- Escape-proof.

- Easy to clean and disinfect.

- Can let light through (transparent) or block light out (opaque).

- Can be worked into almost any shape.

- Lightweight.

- Smooth surfaces means animals are unlikely to cut themselves.

Disadvantages

- Can be less resistant to scratches and bites than metal and glass.

Structure and design

The choice of material will depend on the design of the structure. Considerations will include:

- Portability - is the shelter going to stay in same place or be moved around?

- Weight - is there a maximum and minimum or ideal weight? This is of course very important for portable shelters, but is also important for static structures. Will the weight be fully supported? Will the weight be evenly spread?

- Location - where will the shelter be placed? A shelter that is placed within another building will have different requirements than a standalone shelter, for example.

- Sufficient space - animals require enough space to ensure their lives are comfortable. Accommodation needs to be carefully designed with this in mind, bearing in mind the natural behaviour of the species. Whilst there are laws in place that define minimum space requirements, it is good practice to go beyond that.

- Strength - will the structure be strong enough to contain the animal(s) in question?

- Safety, security and access - ensuring an animal's safety is of paramount importance. Will the structure pose any risk to the animal - for instance, could they cut themselves? Is there an elevated section from which they could fall? For smaller animals, is the entire structure securely located and unable to fall or tip over? Will the animals be able to escape? Will a potential predator be able to gain access (for instance, foxes attacking chickens kept outdoors).

- Ease of cleaning - regular and thorough cleaning is required to kill pathogens, such as bacteria and viruses, and reduce the likelihood of disease. Urine and faeces are a source of pathogens and should be removed regularly. It should be easy to gain access and clean all parts of an animal's accommodation because any hard-to-reach sections are likely to harbour pathogens. The shape of the accommodation and materials from which it is made should not make thorough cleaning difficult.

- Weatherproofing and drainage - accommodation placed outside will be exposed to the elements - sun, wind and rain, and a range of temperatures. To provide a comfortable environment it is important to make sure that animals are protected from them - for instance ensuring that there are no leaks when it rains. Over time the elements can also degrade the accommodation materials. Structures should therefore be weatherproof and provide adequate drainage to stop water gathering. Weather-proofing might mean covering the exterior in another material (e.g. a felt roof), or applying a coating (e.g. a weatherproof varnish to wood). Internal drainage may also be needed for larger animals to help remove urine and water when cleaning.

- Waste disposal - as discussed, removing urine and faeces is an important part of infection control. Accommodation design can make this simpler by providing special toilet areas for animals that can be trained to use them. This can allow easy access for cleaning e.g. providing removable trays for smaller animals, or providing compartments or hatches into which waste can be shovelled. Thought also needs to be given to disposal of waste once removed from accommodation. How close and how easy to access are waste disposal bins or services?

- Location of services - animals need access to drinking water at all times, and water will normally be used when cleaning. For these practical reasons accommodation should be near to a tap or other source of water. Water used for cleaning does not have to be drinking water. Electricity will be needed for lighting, heating and any artificial ventilation, so access to either mains electricity, or a local power source, will be needed. Any electrical supplies or devices will need to be kept fully waterproof - any exposure to water poses a serious threat of electrocution of animals and humans.

- Purpose of accommodation - whilst all of the factors discussed are relevant to all accommodation, the precise purpose of animal accommodation will affect its design. For instance domestic accommodation for the family pet, such as a kennel in the garden, will have simpler requirements than commercial breeding kennels with animals for sale, where there will be large numbers of animals. Similarly temporary accommodation, where animals may be left for a short time waiting to be collected, may be smaller and more basic

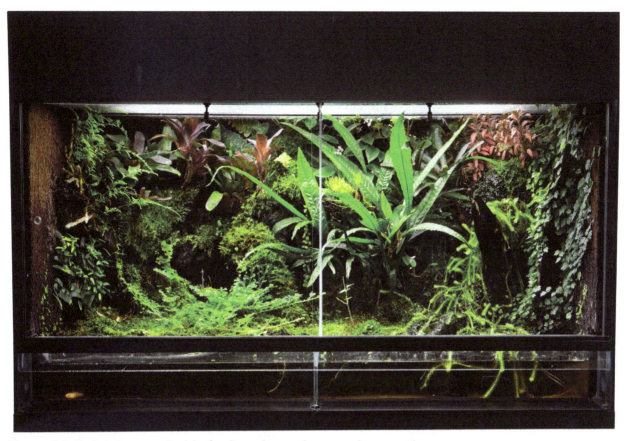

Figure 19 A vivarium - suitable for lizards, snakes or other reptiles

than accommodation designed for long-term housing. Housing in a veterinary surgery has special requirements and there may be several different types - i.e. overnight versus day accommodation, accommodation for animals that need to be isolated, and accommodation for those who have had surgery.

- Suitability for the animals and cost - accommodation for one animal species should of course be perfectly suited to that species' needs. More general accommodation, such as that used in a veterinary surgery, should be designed to be suitable for a range of animals that are commonly treated. If a rare or unusual animal is treated then the accomodation should be assessed with regard to that animal and temporary adaptations made if necessary. Cost is an important factor when designing and building accommmodation and needs to be considered alongside all of the factors previously discussed.

Environmental factors

A number of factors can have a large impact on the comfort and safety of the enviroment in which an animal lives:

- Wind direction - housing should provide animals with shelter from winds. In the UK there is a prevailing south-westerly wind, which means that on average the wind comes from the south-west more often than not. However local geography and conditions play a big part and the prevailing wind may be from a different direction. Any open aspects of housing should not face the prevailing wind.

- Temperature - just like humans, animals are comfortable within a certain range of temperature. That range varies wildly according to species. But, as well as being very uncomfortable and contravening the welfare factors (see next section), an unsuitable temperature can lead to hyperthermia or hypothermia (see Unit 201 section 4.3). Temperature should be carefully and constantly monitored.

- Humidity - this is a measure of how much water vapour is in the air. Warm air can hold more water vapour than cold air, so when temperatures are warm the air can become more humid. (If you are unfamiliar with the idea of humidity, consider how the air feels in a bathroom after a hot shower or bath.) Humid air makes it harder for animals to lose heat; this can be dangerous if they get too hot. It also affects a mammal's perception of temperature - humid conditions at the same temperature as dry conditions will feel warmer. Humid conditions tend to be more uncomfortable for mammals, whereas reptiles from tropical or sub-tropical climates require high humidity. It is therefore important to continually measure humidity as well as temperature. Air conditioning can help to reduce humidity.

- Ventilation - whilst wind and draughts should be avoided, a constant supply of fresh air is vital to stop the buildup of pathogens and remove gases associated with breathing, excreting and the breakdown of food. Ventilation may be natural (through the use of vents, windows etc.) or mechanical (e.g. using an extractor fan or air conditioning).

- Light - animals must be provided both with light, for normal activities, and with a lack of light, for sleeping or other typical behaviour at appropriate times of the day for the species. Whilst natural light is the best option, given the seasonal changes in daylight artificial light may also be needed. Such lights need to be carefully placed to enure an animal cannot poke or chew them. Electrical wires should never be exposed as they pose a very dangerous threat of electrocution. When exposed to natural light, great care should be taken to make sure housing does not warm up to uncomfortable or dangerous levels, and that animals are kept out of direct sunlight on warm days.

- Neighbours - consideration should always be given to residences or businesses that are located nearby. This might be wth regard to noise, light pollution

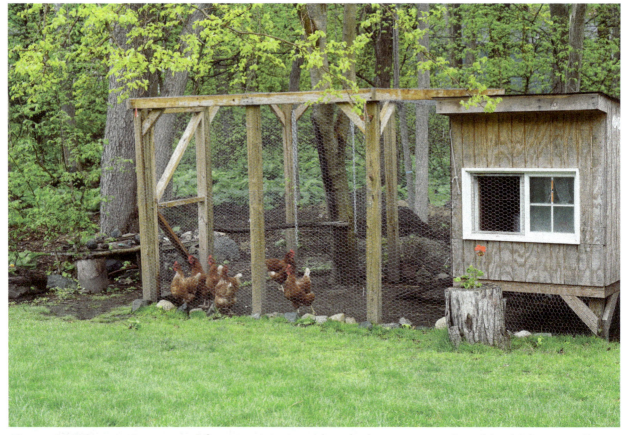

Figure 20 What environmental factors were considered when constructing this chicken coop?

(for instance, an automatic light being activated in the middle of the night), or smells. All of these could be caused by the animals themselves, or by activity related to the animals (for instance food storage, deliveries or other activity). Consideration should also be given as to the effect of human activity on the animals too - for instance being near a factory might disturb or frighten them. When more than one species is being housed careful consideration should be given to how closely they are positioned. The sounds and smells of different species can induce stress in animals that cannot escape. This is particularly true of predatory/prey species.

- Odour pollution - as well as bothering neighbours, unpleasant odours (smells) are undesirable for anyone working with animals. Most smells are due to food or an unclean environment so ensuring uneaten food is cleared away, and keeping the living area very clean, will help to prevent them. Some bedding material is also better at neutralising smells than others. Any muck heaps should be kept well away from buildings and disposed of regularly.

- Waste seepage - animal waste is a source of smells but also a hygiene risk to humans and animals. It is important to ensure it is disposed of correctly and does not leak. Leakage of animal waste will pollute the surrounding environment - a serious health hazard and smells will be impossible to get rid of.

- Noise pollution - animals can be noisy and a group of animals even more so. This can have a negative impact on other animals, people working with them or anyone within earshot. Nocturnal animals, or animals that are not sleeping as normal, can cause a nuisance if they are a source of noise throughout the night. Noise can be reduced through careful positioning of housing, or by using natural sound absorbers such as hedges, bushes or raised mounds of earth. Housing can also be sound-proofed by using cavity walls, sound absorbent tiles,

double-glazing and multiple doors.

Welfare factors

In all work with animals their welfare is the most important factor. All animal housing must therefore conform to the five animal welfare needs that are set out in the Animal Welfare Act 2006. These were covered in Unit 201 section 2.2 but just to recap they are:

- Need for a suitable diet

- Need for a suitable environment

- Need to be able to exhibit normal behaviour patterns

- Need to be housed with, or apart, from other animals

- Need to be protected from pain, suffering, injury and disease

These needs are to be met for all species. It is worth bearing in mind that housing that meets all five needs for one species may not meet them for another species. The needs of each species, and indeed each individual aninal, must be considered when housing them.

The third animal welfare need covers animal behaviour. Behaviour is discussed in more detail in Unit 203. It is an indicator of well-being and must be carefully monitored to ensure that housing and the environment is suitable.

Fixtures and fittings

So far we have discussed the structure and positioning of animal housing. However the content and layout of housing should also be considered.

- Bedding and substrates - bedding refers to the material on which an animal sleeps and substrate is the material which covers the floor. There is further detail on bedding and substrate choices in the next section.

- Hides, beds or boxes - wild animals use their environment to hide from predators, to stalk prey, to hide food and so on. It is not natural for them to be completely exposed and so, when in captivity, there should be spaces provided for them to retreat to. This might be as simple as a box in which they can burrow into bedding or substrate, or a separate hidden section. For much the same reason animals often prefer a separate area to sleep in, and this should be provided.

- Ladders, ramps and levels - following on from the previous point, some animals in the wild will climb their environment. This might be to monitor their surroundings (e.g. a cat sat staring out of a first floor window) or as a way to escape predators. For these species different levels should be provided within their housing, connected by ramps and ladders. This will provide these animals with a more natural and calming environment.

- Natural furnishings - using natural furnishings, such as logs, bushes, trees, plants, grass, water and rocks can help housing to look and feel more like the natural environment in which wild animals live. The extent of natural furnishing will depend on the nature of the housing - for instance, a zoo will have far more requirements than a boarding kennel for dogs. The details also depend, as ever, on the species in question. As well as being benefical for animals, natural furnishings can be used to make the environment more attractive and to blend in with its surroundings, as well as absorb sounds so as to reduce noise pollution.

- Enrichment items - in the wild, animals' daily lives revolve around the search for food and avoiding danger in a complex and ever-changing environment. In captivity food is provided and all danger

is eliminated, and the environment is very simple. This can lead to boredom and depression, which can be detected through atypical behaviour. Enrichment items are used to make the environment more interesting for animals and stop them getting bored. They could take the form of toys such as mirrors or balls, food containers which an animal has to interact with to gain access to contents, or other objects to climb on or interact with, such as swings and tyres.

- Lighting and heating - as discussed a little earlier, animal housing must be lit correctly at the right times of day and kept at the correct temperature, as is appropriate for the species. This may mean heating and lighting needs to be installed within the animal housing. Heating fittings can take the form of radiators, vents, fans or lamps and can be be powered by electricity, oil or gas. Lighting can be in the form of free-standing lamps, ceiling lights or bulbs that are built into walls or ceilings. In all cases the main hazard is that animals interact with the fittings and put themselves or their fellow animals in danger. This might be from chewing electrical cables, burning themselves on a very hot part of a light or heater, or knocking something over. Extreme care must be taken to ensure this cannot happen, regardless of which method of heating or lighting is chosen.

Jargon Buster

substrate material used to cover the floor of animal accommodation

vivarium/terrarium glass cages used to house reptiles carbohydrates

Quiz Questions

1 Give two examples of considerations for accommodation structure and design.

2 Describe three environmental factors that affect animal accommodation.

3 Why might natural furnishings be used in an aviary?

3.2 Prepare animal housing

In this topic you will learn how to prepare suitable housing, fixtures and substrates for species in order to minimise stress and promote animal welfare, considering:

- Species-specific requirements

- Purpose

- Lifestyle

- Life stage

- Number of animals.

You will also learn about different substrate materials, their properties and uses:

- Materials: paper, straw, hay, cardboard, peat, shavings, synthetic bedding, blankets, rubber matting, gravel, sand, soil, vermiculite

Preparing animal housing for selected species

In the previous section we considered the design, structure, materials, environmental factors, fixtures and fittings associated with animal housing. All of these factors should be considered with regard to the five welfare needs, to minimise stress for the animal. In order to do this, you need to consider both the species-specific needs and the needs of the individual animal being housed.

Species-specific requirements
The behaviour and needs of each species will determine the answer to some fundamental questions about the living environment, including:

- socialisation - is the species sociable or solitary?

- neighbours - will other housed animals provide a source of stress? Will wild animals provide a source of stress?

- temperature and humidity - what is a comfortable temperature and humidity range?

- lighting - what level of lighting should be provided and when should lights be on or off?

- space - less space will cause some species more stress than others.

- materials - is the species likely to chew their surroundings, destroying less robust material?

- design - is the species able to climb, or fit through small gaps?

- sleeping - what are their sleeping habits and how does this impact on housing design?

- toileting - what are the species' habits, for instance do they prefer to use one discreet spot? What is the likely impact on cleaning and hygiene?

- enrichment - how much stimulation and enrichment, and of what kind, is helpful for the species in question?

- grooming - does the species require grooming or bathing facilities to be easily accessible?

- security - does the species require extra security measures, for instance because they are dangerous or are simply good at escaping?

Purpose
The purpose of accommodation affects many choices about its design. Different purposes include:

- Kennels and catteries, offering overnight

65

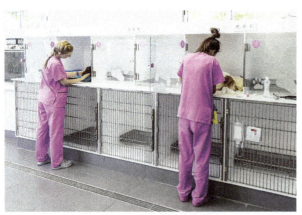 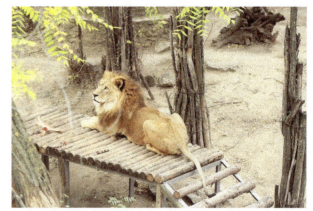

Figure 21 Accommodation in a veterinary surgery has different requirements from that in a zoo

accommodation, normally for a limited amount of time for each animal.

- Breeding kennels.

- Rescue centres where animals may be housed in the short, medium or long term.

- Accommodation for working animals.

- A zoo, where they would expect to spend a majority of their time within accommodation, but allowing the general public to observe them

- Farms, where the business of running a farming opertion is another factor that needs to be taken into account.

- Short-term accommodation for trading and selling animals.

- Companion animals, where the purpose is simply to house animals comfortably.

Within a veterinary surgery there are different types of housing:

- Overnight accommodation for animals who are sick.

- Post-surgery special-care accommodation for animals recently out of surgery or who are very ill.

- Day accommodation for animals who have been treated for minor conditions and are simply waiting for their owner.

The purpose will affect some of the factors we have discussed. For instance, ease of cleaning and hygienic procedures will be critical in a veterinary surgery, whilst neighbouring species will have to be very carefully considered in a zoo.

Lifestyle and life stage

Lifestyle and life stage will also impact decisions on housing. For instance:

- Sedentary or active - species that are naturally active will require more space than those which are less active, assuming that they spend most of their time within the housing environment.

- Working or farm animal - working animals may spend a great deal of time away from their housing environment in which case it can be simpler as they will receive stimulation and exercise elsewhere. Farm animals may spend a great deal of time in their housing environment but equally they may require access to pasture or outdoor areas. These details may change over the course of a year.

- Companion animals - exotic and smaller companion animals may spend all of their time within the housing environment whereas cats and dogs are often not housed separately at all and share the living space with their owners.

- Sick, ill and injured animals - animals that are ill or injured may have special requirements including different temperatures, better ventilation and the elimination of stress. They are likely to be kept separate and particular attention given to cleaning and disinfection of their living area.

- Juvenile - young animals are particularly playful with a great deal of energy. Consideration of this should be made with regard to other animals around them. It may also be appropriate for a solitary species to live together socially when young.

- Old age - older (geriatric) animals tend to sleep more and be less active. They are likely to prefer calmer environments and reduced levels of stress.

- Breeding, pregnant or lactating animals - the behaviour of breeding animals, both male and female, is different to normal which might require special temporary changes to accommodation - for instance, keeping adult males away from each other. In the later stages of pregnancy the female may need to be isolated to reduce the risk of infection and reduce any chance of aggression with another animal, both of which could result in a miscarriage, though this depends on the species. Some species may prefer a box to give birth in, from which the newborns cannot escape. Young animals often need to be kept isolated from other adults apart from their mother. Environmental conditions may need adjusting, according to species, during the milking phase for mammals.

Number of animals

The number of animals must be considered in line with the five welfare needs. Some species may need to be completely solitary and distant, whereas other species may require them to form social groups. Too many animals in too small a space is a source of stress for any species however, so you must carefully research recommended guidelines for the species you are working with.

Identification and selection of different types of substrate

There are a range of different materials that can be used as substrates for different species. Substrates should keep the animal warm, be able to absorb or drain away urine and other liquids but prevent the build-up of smells. They should also be safe, with no sharp edges, and should not contain harmful bacteria or dust mites that cause allergic reactions that lead to breathing issues. Materials that do not cause allergic reactions are called hypoallergenic. It must, of course, also be safe for the animal to walk on the substrate.

Straw, hay and shavings

Straw resembles hay but is yellow/brown in colour, is a by-product of harvesting cereal crops and has low nutritional value. This may or may not be a good thing, depending on the animal, but it is therefore very cheap.

Both straw and hay are relatively absorbent and insulating, and are often used in livestock animals' pens and stables. They can also be used for smaller companion animals though they can be too rough for smaller animals.

Wood shavings can also be used for livestock and companion animals but care must be taken to ensure that they are not sharp or liable to splinter. It is recommended to only use wood shavings that have been treated specifically for animal use.

Straw, hay and shavings can all harbour dust mites which can cause allergic reactions in susceptible animals.

Paper and cardboard

Paper and cardboard sheets can be used to line living areas as they have some absorbent and insulating properties. As they are from recycled sources, and will biodegrade, they are environmentally friendly. However the inks used for printing can be poisonous so care must be taken when choosing paper. Glossy paper used in magazines is not suitable. If they get too wet then they can become slippy, so it's often a good idea to use them together with another substrate material.

Instead of sheets, shredded paper can be used instead. This might be more suitable for small companion animals.

Peat and soil

Peat is an organic material formed from the partial decomposition of plants in damp conditions without any oxygen. Once cut and dried, peat is very absorbent and insulating.

67

Both peat and soil may be used for reptiles and other exotic animals. Commercially available soil is treated before use - it is not safe to use soil from the garden for such animals.

Gravel, sand and vermiculite

Vermiculite is a mineral that is suitable for use with insects and reptiles.

All three of these allow liquid to drain through them rather than absorb them. This can be an advantage as long as the liquid has somewhere to drain to underneath.

Synthetic bedding, blankets, rubber mats

Synthetic bedding can be easier to work with and keep clean but may not be as comfortable as natural materials. It is also possible, or even very likely, that an animal will chew or eat the material so it must be completely non-toxic and not pose a choking hazard.

Blankets can be used to keep animals warm, and are absorbent. They must be kept clean but are easy to wash.

Rubber mats are often used to line horses' stables as they are good insulators and provide support for the animal's limbs.

Rubber is not absorbent but interlocking mats can be designed to allow liquids to drain to the level below. Rubber mats are often used with some other substrate material.

Substrate uses

Substrates are used to make the environment more comfortable for the animal. For animals who will spend most or all of their time within their housing environment, substrates can be used to enrich that environment, giving the animal something interesting to explore. With this in mind, peat, soil and gravel can be used to grow plants or other organic material. Such plants, along with the substrate itself, can help to simulate the natural outdoor environment in which the animal is normally found.

More than one substrate can be used within an animal's accommodation, either in layers on top of each other or placed in zones. The former allows you to use the best properties of each substrate whereas the latter helps to keep the environment interesting and minimise the negative aspects of any substrate.

Overleaf is a summary of some substrate properties.

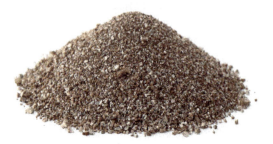

Figure 22 Vermiculite

Jargon Buster

sedentary inactive

lactating producing milk

hypoallergenic a term meaning something that does not cause allergic reactions

biodegrade to break down naturally in the environment

vermiculite a mineral used as a bedding material

Quiz Questions

1 Give two examples of different types of accommodation and describe the differences between them.

2 List a) a suitable substrate for an animal with known allergies, b) an unsuitable substrate for the same animal. Justify your answers.

3 What special accommodation requirements might a new mother have?

Material	Insulation	Absorption	Hypo-allergenic	Odour contol	Durability	Bio-degradable	Non-slip
Paper	Good	Fair	Yes	Poor	Poor	Yes	No
Straw	Good	Good	No	Poor	Poor	Yes	No
Hay	Good	Good	No	Poor	Poor	Yes	No
Cardboard	Good	Good	Yes	Poor	Poor	Yes	No
Peat	Very good	Good	Yes	Good	Poor	Yes	Yes
Shavings	Good	Good	No	Good	Poor	Yes	Yes
Synthetic bedding	Good	Fair	Yes	Fair	Good	No	Yes
Blankets	Very good	Good	Yes	Poor	Good	No	Yes
Rubber matting	Very good	Poor	Yes	Poor	Good	No	Yes
Gravel	Poor	Poor	Yes	Poor	Good	No	Yes
Sand	Poor	Poor	Yes	Poor	Good	No	Yes
Soil	Fair	Good	Yes	Poor	Good	Yes	Yes
Vermiculite	Good	Poor	Yes	Good	Good	No	Yes

3.3 Clean animal housing

In this topic you will learn about the preparation and cleaning routines of animal accommodation and the disposal of waste in accordance with legislation and industry good practice standards:

- **Preparation of cleaning**

- **Cleaning routines and frequencies**

- **Factors influencing changes to cleaning routines and frequency of cleaning**

- **The need for safe cleaning to include safe working practices and legislation**

- **Safe disposal of waste**

It is very important to keep animal housing clean. This is because pathogens such as bacteria and viruses, which cause diseases, breed in dirty conditions. Cleaning prevents this by:

- killing pathogens

- removing the material on which pathogens live - for instance, fur, faeces and urine.

Preparation of cleaning

Use of Personal Protective Equipment (PPE)

Personal Protective Equipment refers to any item which keeps the user safe from hazards. When it comes to cleaning animals housing there are two main risks:

- Contact with animal waste that contains pathogens. These pathogens are dangerous because some diseases are zoonotic which means they can be passed from animals to humans. Some zoonotic diseases are very dangerous or even fatal. The best way to prevent them is to avoid any contact with pathogens in the first place.

- Contact with, or inhalation of, the cleaning products themselves. There are many different products but some chemicals used to clean dirt and kill pathogens can irritate the skin or sensitive areas of the body such as eyes and lungs.

PPE for cleaning often takes the form of rubber gloves, gowns, boots and goggles. Equipment should be specially designed for use as PPE - for instance you should not use normal fabric gloves.

All PPE should fit correctly and not inhibit movement or increase other risks (for instance, by tripping over ill-fitting boots).

PPE should only be worn for cleaning, and then stored separately from non-PPE equipment, to avoid cross-contamination.

Reusable PPE equipment should also be cleaned regularly, using antisceptic wipes or by washing - again, this should be done separately from non-PPE equipment. Disposable PPE should diposed of after use.

Selection of cleaning equipment

Typical cleaning equipment would include:

- cloths and hand brushes - used to disinfect and scrub surfaces

- shovels - to remove large amounts of waste material

- mops - used to clean and disinfect floors

- buckets - used to store disinfectant and detergent, and to rinse dirty cloths, brushes and mops

- measuring equipment - if the buckets do not measure the amount of liquid in them then separate measuring buckets may be needed when diluting cleaning products

- sponges - used to absorb excess water

- dustpan and brush - used to remove

dust, hair and other dry material before cleaning with detergent and disinfectant

- bin bags - for disposal of solid waste

- vacuum cleaners - also used to remove dry material, they can be quicker and limit the spread of material; however the same appliance must not be used for domestic purposes and its contents must be disposed of as contaminated waste

- high-pressure hose - used for larger housing which would take a long time to wash by hand

- steam cleaners - instead of hot water, these boil water to generate steam at an even higher temperature; the high temperature itself helps to kill pathogens; steam cleaners are particularly useful for cleaning fabrics.

Use of a holding tank/cage/stable/ stall/pen

As discussed, some cleaning products are hazardous and they present a risk to animals as well as humans. Animals should be removed from their normal housing before cleaning begins - in fact, for some cleaning products it is essential that they are removed. It is also much easier to clean without animals present!

Animals can be placed in temporary accommodation whilst their normal housing is cleaned. Because it is temporary it can be smaller and less perfectly suited to them. However if the cleaning operation is likely to take a long time then a better standard of temporary accommodation should be provided.

Correct dilution of cleaning agents and disinfectants

There are different classes of cleaning products that perform different functions:

- a detergent is the name for a broad family of cleaning agents that essentially enables grease and oil to mix with water, and therefore be washed away with water.

- A disinfectant is a broad term for a family of chemicals that is designed to kill pathogens on surfaces. Different disinfectants may be designed to kill different pathogens, or they may be more general. If there is a risk of a particular disease, caused by specfic pathogens, then the most appropriate disinfectant should be selected. Disinfectants contain hazardous chemicals that are dangerous for humans and animals.

Given the wide range of different cleaning products, made up of a wide range of different potentially hazardous chemicals, the most important thing to do before any cleaning begins is to read the manufacturer's instructions. These should be followed very carefully, to avoid harm and injury.

Some cleaning products may be in a concentrated form and may require dilution before application. Dilution means mixing with another substance - normally water. It is very important that the dilution instructions are followed exactly as stated, because the chemicals may be unsafe to use in their concentrated form. For instance, instead of simply irritating the skin when diluted, they may actually burn the skin when concentrated. If the product is diluted with too much water then it may not work properly.

Dilution instructions are often something like:

"Mix one capful of cleaning product with five litres of water before application."

In this case, five litres of water should be carefully measured out before adding the cap of cleaning product.

Note that it is the ratio of cleaning product to amount of water that is important. So, using this example, if you needed to clean a large area that required ten litres of water, then you would add two capfuls - i.e. you would multiply the amount of cleaning product AND water by two.

Similarly, if you were cleaning a smaller area, and only required 2.5 litres of water, then you would add half a capful - i.e. you would use half the amount of cleaning fluid AND half the amount of water.

Warm or hot water can help the cleaning product to be more effective - the instructions will state the ideal temperature of the water.

Cleaning routines and frequencies

Full and spot cleaning

A full clean is when all surfaces within the animal's housing are fully cleaned and disinfected. Normal practice depends on species and setting but a full clean would be carried out at least once per week. If a lot of animals share the same space then a full clean might be needed more often.

A typical full cleaning routine would be:

- remove animals to a holding area or alternative accommodation

- remove objects and equipment, such as water bowls and bedding, from the accommodation.

- remove all organic material, such as faeces and urine

- sweep or vaccum to remove hair and fur, and then wash away any that remains

- use a detergent with warm water to fully clean the area, using brushes, mops and cloths as appropriate, and then rinse away

- apply disinfectant and leave it for as long as the manufacturer recommends, making sure all surfaces are covered including those that are hard to reach or out of sight

- rinse away, making sure no disinfectant remains

- leave until fully dry before reintroducing equipment and animals.

A spot clean is focused on a smaller area of accommodation and equipment. Spot clean of high-use areas and equipment should be carried out at least once per day. Further spot cleans may be required due to one-off events such as an animal vomiting, so they are carried out whenever they are required.

Water changes

Water is likely to become contaminated with food, bedding, fur or hair, and faeces over time. This is particularly true when multiple animals use the same water. Dirty water is a

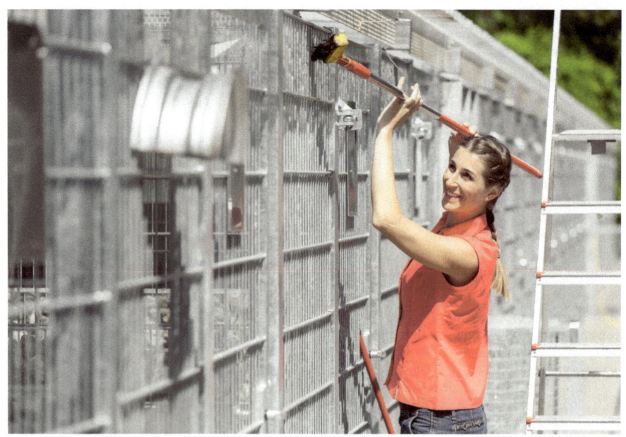

Figure 23 It is important to keep living areas clean

major health hazard and therefore fresh, clean water should be provided throughout the day. If containers are open to contamination then they should be cleaned during the day too.

Water that is left within a bowl during a full cleaning process will become contaminated with cleaning products which are poisonous. Like all surfaces, feeding and water bowls should be thoroughly rinsed out after cleaning, to make sure there is no trace of cleaning product left.

Disinfection

Disinfectants work best when dirt and animal substances have already been removed. In fact some disinfectants will not work at all if organic material is present. This means that fur, hair and other large material should be swept or vacuumed away first, and then surfaces cleaned with detergent to remove dirt, grease and oil. Only once that has been done should disinfectant should be applied. It **must** then be left in contact with the surface, in line with the manufacturer's instructions. This is very important because rinsing it away immediately may allow pathogens to survive.

If more than one disinfectant is used, in order to target different pathogens, then each should be applied, rinsed and dried before applying the next one.

Once disinfectant has been thoroughly rinsed then surfaces should be left to dry. Note that disinfectants are poisonous, so animals must not be present when applying. For the same reason, it must be fully rinsed away after use.

When using a new disinfectant, it should be tested on a small area of the surface to be cleaned, to make sure that it does not damage the material.

Factors influencing changes to cleaning routines and frequency

Prior to and after birthing, and early lactation

Mothers will often want to find a quiet place to give birth in. You should ensure that this spot is clean and disinfected before the female enters. As birth approaches the mother may be unwilling to move for normal cleaning

72

routines, so you might need to line the birthing area with paper, bedding or other easy-to-remove substrates.These should then be removed and replaced with clean ones daily.

The birth itself will produce fluids and tissue that will need to be removed and cleaned up. In mammals, the mother will normally clean the newborn animals but she herself may need cleaning where she is, using a soft sponge or cloth.

Newborn mammals have some level of immunity passed on from their mother - however both theirs and their mother's immune system will be relatively weak and open to infection. Reducing exposure to pathogens through cleaning will help protect them.

In the days after birth, mammalian mothers are unlikely to want to leave their offspring and it is not a good idea to try to move them. So blankets, newspapers and other temporary bedding should continue to be replaced each day. Normal cleaning routines should only resume once mother and offspring are happy being moved.

The newborn animals will not be toilet trained during the early lactation stage. So the living area will continue to need cleaning on a regular basis. Once they begin to explore their environment and venture away from their mother, you can begin to think about returning to normal cleaning routines.

After surgery

Animals recovering from surgery will be weakened, with a less effective immune system. They will also have wounds, which are another way in with pathogens can enter the body. Their accommodation must, therefore, be completely disinfected before they arrive.

Once they are in place their accommodation should be cleaned and disinfected as regularly as possible but with minimal disruption to the patient who will be uncomfortable or in pain.

The patient should be kept away from other animals and equipment should not be shared between them.

Following similar guidlines as for contagious

diseases, below, will reduce the risk of infection.

Gravely ill

Very ill animals have weakend immune systems and are more susceptible to disease than normal. Catching another disease when already ill can be fatal, so their environment needs to be throughly disinfected. They may be less able or willing to move than normal so more spot cleaning of equipment may be required.

Contagious illness

Contagious diseases can be passed on to other animals. Therefore animals with symptoms of these diseases need to be isolated from other animals. Special measures need to be put in place to prevent cross contamination - these measures are collectively known as barrier nursing. They include:

- a limited number of people should interact with the infected animals

- an outer layer of clothes which are only used when cleaning the infected area

- cleaning and PPE equipment used to clean the infected animal's accommodation must not be moved to, or used, in any other area

- careful disposal of any waste in separate containers

- very careful attention must be paid to ensure the cleaner themselves does not transmit the disease - this means that thorough hand-washing routines using appropriate antisceptics are in place, even if gloves are worn.

- even after cleaning, equipment such as bedding, food bowls etc. should not be shared between contagious and non-contagious animals.

- in a cleaning routine, infectious animals should be cleaned last.

Zoonotic illness

A zoonotic disease is one that can be passed from animals to humans. This means that the

73

cleaner is at risk. Therefore appropriate action must be taken to minimise this risk.

To protect against human infection, the method of transmission of the zoonotic disease must be understood. For instance, if transmission was airborne then the PPE equipment would need to include a mask. If the pathogens could live on any surface then it would be sensible to use a spray disinfectant to minimise the touching of surfaces.

Measures to protect against zoonotic diseases would therefore be similar to those for contagious illness, except extra steps should be in place to ensure that infected equipment is handled by as few people as possible; and those people also follow strict hygiene rules.

The need for safe cleaning to include safe working practices and legislation

Health and Safety at Work Act (1974)

This Act spells out the responsibilities that employers and employees have to keep their workplaces safe.

For employers this means they must:

- provide all relevant equipment to keep safe (for instance, gloves to use when handling disinfectants)

- provide training on how to use equipment properly

- maintain equipment in good working order, and store materials and equipment in a safe manner

- conduct risk assessments of all activities to identify potential hazards and then take measures to reduce the chance of any accidents, through training and by implementing systems of work

- have a formal written health and safey policy.

In the context of cleaning, as well as covering cleaning activities themselves, risk assessments would also cover potential risks when moving animals.

For employees, they must:

- follow the health and safety policy of the organisation and put into practice any health and safety training they have received

- report any damaged or missing equipment

- report any hazards or potential hazards that they see.

In the context of cleaning this might mean, for instance, that you notice the water from a hot tap is dangerously hot and presents a burn risk, or that the gloves you have been given have holes in, potentially exposing skin to cleaning products.

The Reporting of Injuries, Diseases and Dangerous Occurrences Regulations (2013) (RIDDOR)

These regulations cover any incident defined as an injury, disease or dangerous occurence.

An injury is defined as an event that causes some physical trauma and includes:

- burns

- damage to the eye

- lung damage or breathing problems

- any injury which causes someone to be off work for seven days or more.

Diseases that are likely to have been caused by work must also be reported, for instance:

- asthma

- tendonitis.

Dangerous occurences are specifically defined within the regulations but cover things like the release of toxic chemicals, explosions, collapsing structures, and electrical fires.

All such cases must be reported to the Health and Safety Executive, even if injury was avoided.

Control of Substances Hazardous to Health Regulations (2002) (COSHH) and centre risk assessments

These regulations require employers to control the use of any substance which poses a health hazard, and have measures in places to minimise risks. The requirements include:

- conduct risk assessments to understand the health risks associated with the substance and put measures in place to reduce those risks

- control access to hazardous substances (for instance, by storing substances in a secure area with limited access)

- provide training to all relevant members of staff when handling substances

- provide PPE and training on how to use it

- have response plans in place in case of emergency

The COSHH regulations cover the products used for cleaning and disinfecting.

Animal Welfare Act 2006

Covered in Unit 201 section 2.1, this Act is in place to ensure all animals' welfare needs are being met and that they are not being mistreated. With regard to cleaning practices, the points that are particularly relevant are:

- animals are housed in a suitable environment (place to live)

- animals are free of 'pain, injury, suffering and disease'.

This means that housing should be clean, free of pathogens which cause disease, and are safe - i.e. they are not exposed to toxic detergents and disinfectants.

Safe disposal of waste

Hazardous and non-hazardous waste

Organisations working with animals produce waste that is hazardous to human health. Even waste that is not hazardous can be unpleasant. This has led to strict rules about

how to dispose of waste, governed by the Environmental Protection Act 1990.

Hazardous waste is made up of of the following:

- Infectious clinical waste: any bodily fluids, organs, and any material that is contaminated with these substances.

- Cytotoxic medicines: these are medicines that are toxic to human cells - they are used to treat conditions such as cancer but are hazardous to handle. All such medicines, including unused or partly-used medicines, tablets, containers etc. should be disposed of separately to other waste.

- Contaminated sharps: scalpels, scissors, syringes and other equipment used to perform medical procedures that have been contaminated with bodily fluids should be disposed of separately to unused sharps.

Non-hazardous waste is made up of:

- Offensive waste: this includes faeces, wipes, cloths and disposable PPE that has not been contaminated with infectious material.

- Dead animals: as long as there is no suspicion that the body contains an infectious disease, bodies can be transferred to owners for burial or cremation; otherwise they are disposed of with the infectious clinical waste.

- Non-contaminated sharps.

- Non-cytotoxic medicines.

- Domestic waste: such as packaging, food etc.

Good environmental practices

Every person, business and organisation has a part to play in protecting our environment. In practice this means reducing, re-using and recycling wherever possible. Organisations that work with animals can help by:

- **Composting.** This means encouraging organic material, such as wasted food, to break down naturally to form compost that can be used as fertiliser. Faeces from

75

vegetarian animals can also be used for this purpose. Compost could be created on-site, or the waste could be separated out and collected by a third party.

- **Recycling**. Plastics, paper, cardboard, glass, cans and other material can be recyled into new products. This cuts down on landfill and also decreases the need for new raw materials. Recycling facilities are available in most places and simply requires recylable material to be separated out.

Preventing cross-contamination

Given that waste is broadly classified as hazardous or non-hazardous, it is very important that non-hazardous waste is not contaminated by hazardous waste. If it were, then people handling waste would be put at risk.

To make sure this does not happen, a system of colour-coded bins and bags are used for each of the main categories of waste. This allows for them to be collected separately so they can then be disposed of in a safe way.

It is good practice for the waste bins to be kept in a secure area, with access limited to authorised people. This will help prevent waste being placed in the incorrect bin.

Jargon Buster

cytotoxic substances that kill animal cells

detergent a chemical used to clean away dirt

disinfectant a chemical used to kill pathogens

zoonotic a disease that can pass from animal to human

barrier nursing a method of preventing cross-contamination

antisceptic a substance similar to a disinfectant but which is suitable for use on skin

Quiz Questions

1 Describe the differences between a detergent and a disinfectant.

2 Outline the differences between a full clean and a spot clean.

3 Name two pieces of legislation that are relevant to cleaning working practices.

4 Describe the differences between hazardous and non-hazardous waste.

LO4 Maintain animal accommodation

4.1 Safety and security checks on animal housing

4.2 Maintain animal housing

In these topics you will learn about safety and security checks and the reasons for them:

• To ensure the safety of the animal(s), self and others

• Prevent escape or unwanted breeding.

You will also learn how to recognise and report basic animal housing maintenance, and the basic tools needed for maintenance, spare equipment (screws, nails, wire mesh, light bulbs, fixtures and fittings).

Safety and security checks

Animal accommodation must be checked regulary to make sure it is safe and escape-proof.

The structure itself, and the equipment contained within it, must be kept safe for both animals and people. Potential hazards might include:

• broken glass

• slip hazard from a spillage

• sharp edges or exposed splinters caused by animals gnawing

Housing must also be checked to make sure that animals cannot escape and wild animals cannot enter. This would include checking that all locks, doors, windows and any other openings, are all in good working order. For instance, a wooden window frame that fitted perfectly in the winter may begin to stick in the summer.

If the housing has a fence then the entire fence must be checked for damage or missing sections. Bear in mind that such damage may be on the outside if caused by wild animals.

The same checks are needed if animals are separated within housing, for instance if males and females are kept away from each other to prevent breeding, or mothers and new-born offspring are isolated for their safety and comfort.

Safety and security checks need to be carried out regularly and reported in order to be fixed. A serious safety or security issue should be reported immediately.

Basic animal housing maintenance

Over time animal housing will need small repairs and maintenance. These basic repairs can be done by anyone with some training and understanding.

To perform repairs and maintenance you will need access to some basic tools such as:

• hammer

• screwdriver

• scalpel or knife

• masking tape

• saw

• sandpaper

You will also need some equipment and fittings, such as:

• nails and screws

• wire mesh

• light bulbs

- any other replacement fittings that are used in the accommodation.

As this is a practical topic you will be shown how these tools can be used to perform basic repairs and maintenance including:

- replacement or repair of damaged security and locks - this is obviously an important security task

- damaged wooden structures - this may or may not be a critical repair, depending on the location

- protruding nails

- cracked glass - this can be both a safety and security hazard

- broken/bent wire - normally in a fence or a cage

- blown light or heat bulb

- replacement of filter pads - used in aquariums

- breakage of loose fixtures and fittings - the exact details will depend on the fixture or fitting in question.

Quiz Questions

1 Name two things that a safety check should cover.

2 Describe two maintenance tasks that you could be asked to carry out and why they would be needed.

Unit 203 Animal behaviour and handling

LO1 Recognise the difference between normal and atypical behaviour

In these topics you will learn how to identify the following typical behaviours of your selected species through observation:

- Eating, drinking, movement, sleeping patterns, visual and auditory intraspecific communication, social behaviour

You will also learn how to recognise atypical behaviours and their cause:

- Fear, aggression and stress-related behaviour

1.1 Behaviour in animals

Observation of selected species to identify typical behaviours

In the wild each animal species has certain patterns of behaviour. This behaviour has evolved over tens of thousands of years and is considered typical for that species.

Domesticated animals and pets have evolved from wild animals and have inherited many patterns of behaviour from their ancestors. As a result they also display behaviour which is considered typical for their species.

It is important that you are able to observe and understand typical behaviour for your chosen species.

Eating and drinking

When it comes to eating, animals fall into three main categories:

- carnivores
- herbivores
- omnivores.

Carnivores must eat meat for nutritional reasons, and act as predators to survive. The larger the animals they typically prey on, the less often they have to eat but the more effort required to kill. This might mean that, in captivity, feeding is less frequent than for other animals, as their digestion is designed to take on large amounts of food at irregular periods - for instance, snakes.

Other carnivores are scavengers, eating meat from animals that they have not themselves killed. This may be leftovers from predators or animals that have died from natural, or human, causes. They are more likely to eat irregularly as they are dependent on circumstances.

Herbivores do not require meat to survive. They are more likely to forage for food such as grass, plants, seeds, nuts and fruit. Herbivores are likely to eat smaller amounts of food more regularly than carnivores.

Omnivores are animals that can survive eating plant material or meat. They can adapt to eating either.

Other behaviour associated with eating includes:

- sharing food with a group / not sharing

and being protective or even aggressive over food

- eating in the open or eating while hidden

- hiding or storing food to be eaten later - either the next few days or over an extended period such as winter

- feeding times can differ across species - nocturnal animals will of course feed during their active hours at night.

Movement

Animals are at their most and least active at different times of the day and will vary by species.

Natural patterns of movement in wild animals are mainly determined by their methods of finding food and avoiding being eaten. For instance:

- Predator species may roam to find prey or keep to the same location and lay in wait. They may have sudden short bursts of energy when going in for a kill but otherwise be fairly inactive. Over time, in the search for food in the wild, they may slowly roam over large areas.

- Foraging species are more likely to be active for longer periods of the day, constantly looking for food and eating. They will move slowly covering ground as they feed.

Domestic animals will inherit behaviour from their wild ancestors but have also been bred by humans to promote certain characteristics. This means that different breeds will display different behaviours:

- Dogs have evolved from a predator species and display some movements that are natural for a hunter. Some breeds, such as beagles, make use of this and have been bred for hunting. Their natural instincts will be to follow a scent and will require plenty of exercise.

- Cats are natural hunters. They will establish a territory which they will patrol at their most active times of the day. This may be quite a large area - but they are likely to be inactive for the other parts of the day.

Livestock animals have been domesticated but behave like foragers if given the space, grazing for many hours a day and slowly moving around fields or paddocks.

Exotic animals such as reptiles exhibit different kinds of behaviour. Many species are fairly inactive but there are exceptions- tortoises, turtles, and certain breeds of lizard. Activity levels in reptiles depend on the temperature - if it is too cold they may stop moving for an extended period of time.

Sleeping patterns

This differs greatly across different species - so make sure you research what is typical for your chosen species.

Some examples of sleeping patterns:

- Many animals, including humans, are diurnal - that is, they are awake during the day and sleep at night.

- However, some animals are nocturnal - this means they sleep during the day and wake at night, e.g. hamsters.

- Other animals are crepuscular - this means they are most active at dawn and dusk, and sleep at other times. Examples include cats, rodents and rabbits.

- Dogs will sleep for hours at a time across different times of the day, and may spend around 12 hours asleep each day – although this depends on species, age and the individual animal.

- Cats can sleep from 12-16 hours a day, although that tends to be a light sleep so they can react to any perceived threat. They are most active at dawn and dusk

- Whilst birds can sleep normally they are also able to sleep with only one half of the brain at a time. This allows them to keep one eye open and alert whilst partly asleep. If the right-hand part of the brain is asleep then the left eye can be kept open and vice versa.

- Horses sleep standing up, for about three hours per day.

- Cows and sheep will sleep lying down if they are comfortable and safe in their surroundings, for about four hours per day.

- Pigs sleep lying down for about eight hours per day.

Visual and auditory intraspecific communication

Intraspecific communication means communication betweeen the same species.

Visual communication

Animals (and humans) communicate how they are feeling through their body language and facial expressions. For instance, a dog can adopt a number of different postures according to how it feels (Figure 24):

- Alert – tail up, ears forward, closed mouth, raised up on paws.

- Dominant aggressive – tail up and large, ears forward, mouth open and lips curled, baring teeth, raised hackles.

- Fearful – tail down, ears back, lowered body.

- Happy or playful – tail up or wagging, ears up, mouth open, crouching down with front paws.

Similarly, a cat will also communicate its mood and behaviour through its posture (Figure 25):

- Alert – ears up, sat up straight, tail on the floor possibly moving slowly back and forth.

- Aggressive – tail up and bushy, ears down, fur stood up, arched back, mouth open.

- Fearful – crouched down, muscles tense, tail tucked away, dilated pupils.

- Happy or playful – tail up and curled, closed mouth, standing in a relaxed posture. A cat that is feeling happy and trusts you will expose its belly.

There are many more different moods that can be communicated with subtle differences in posture and movement.

There are differences between cats and dogs in the meaning of their body language. It is unsurprising that the two species can find it hard to interpret each other's moods and intentions and do not always get on.

Whilst humans have the most expressive faces, with a reported 27 different facial expressions, animals can also display different emotions with different expressions. Socialised animals have more expressions, and animals like dogs, cats and horses have numerous different expressions. Chimpanzees also have very expressive faces. Some of the characteristics of these expressions are similar across different species, for example:

- wide eyes often demonstrate an alert state

- piercing, hard stares often are a sign of agitation or a direct challenge

- baring teeth, unsurprisingly, is often a sign of aggression

- yawning when not tired can be a sign of stress.

Auditory communication

Auditory is another word for sound. Sounds are a useful form of communication because they can transmit information over large distances. The sounds that animals make to communicate can either be made with the voice or with other parts of their body. Much auditory communication is concerned with finding or locating food, finding a mate, fending off predators or warning off rivals. Vocal sounds include:

- barking – used by dogs to alert other members of the pack to a potential threat but is likely to be used to communicate other information too

- growling, hissing, roaring – normally a warning sound

- purring – communicates pleasure or contentment

- howling – used for a range of reasons e.g. marking territory

- whimpering – can be associated with submission

- singing – used by birds and whales to

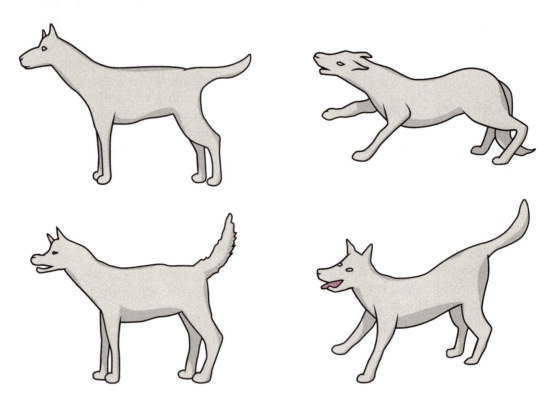

Figure 24 Body language of a dog: a) alert (top left) b) fearful (top right) c) dominant aggressive (bottom left), d) happy or playful (bottom right)

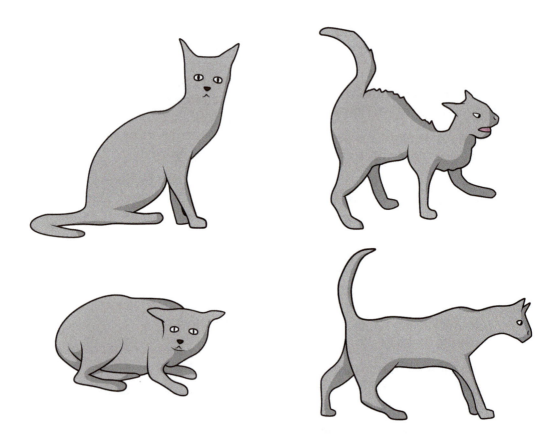

Figure 25 Body language of a cat: a) alert (top left) b) aggressive (top right) c) fearful (bottom left) d) happy or playful (bottom right)

define their territory and for attracting mates

- vocalisations are often used as a method of communication between mothers and new-born offspring.

There are many other examples across lots of different species. Some, like the songs of humpback whales, are very complex and sophisticated – so sophisticated in fact that there is some evidence of differing dialects in different areas.

Non-vocal communication examples include:

- 'chirping' of crickets and grasshoppers – his sound is made when crickets rub their wings together, and when a grasshopper rubs its wing with its leg

- the sound of the rattlesnake, made by shaking the distinctive end of their tail

- the slap of a dolphin tail on the surface of the sea

- gorillas beating their chest.

Social behaviour

Social behaviour refers to the way in which animals interact with each other. These interactions may be for a range of different reasons, for instance:

- to find food

- to find shelter

- to find a mate.

Some behaviours may be shared across different species – for instance mammals – whereas others may be species-specific. Even within a species different breeds may be more or less sociable. Individual animals will also have their own tendencies too.

- Social units may consist of a full group (e.g. wolf packs or a pride of lions), a pair of adults of the opposite sex (such as is the case with many bird species), or solitary adults (e.g. various big cats in the wild).

- Feral cats form social groups because they benefit from sharing food and there is safety in numbers. For domestic cats food is not in short supply and they are not

in any danger, so they have a tendency towards solitary behaviour. However, they can still form social groups. When domestic cats are in the same social group you will see them grooming each other and sleeping together. If they are not part of the same social group then multiple cats in one house may regard each other as rivals, which may or may not lead to aggression. Cats can be aggressive with other cats who do not live with them who appear in their territory.

- Dogs are social animals, which means that they do not like to be by themselves and seek out the company of familiar dogs or humans. This means that they need to be able to understand social signals. Dogs learn to predict how other dogs and humans will behave in certain situations, which then influences their own behaviour.

- Dogs will behave differently with strange dogs compared to familiar dogs, as each tries to establish how the other dog will react. Strange dogs will approach each other with some caution and each may be naturally friendly, playful, aggressive, fearful etc. But regardless of that, each dog will try to predict the other's behaviour and react in a way that it thinks best.

- Typical social behaviour of dogs includes: barking, to warn other members of the family about intruders or potential danger; play-fighting; smelling each other to establish mood and behaviour; sleeping together; greeting returning members of the family.

- Other animals that like the company of their species include: horses, donkeys, cows, pigs, sheep, goats, chickens, gerbils, mice and rats.

- Common solitary animals include hamsters and most reptiles.

Dominance and submission

In social groups animals will form relationships with each other. For some species a pair of animals will form a dominant and submissive relationship. This means that the submissive animal will give way to the dominant animal.

When animals live in groups of more than two, all of the different dominant-submissive relationships can become quite complex. However their purpose is to allow groups to live together peacefully because each animal knows how it should behave to another. This prevents constant fighting and aggression over food and other resources.

All sorts of factors can play a part in why one animal is dominant over another – this includes size/weight, age, sex, breed, and certain anatomical features or displays.

Animals use different methods of communication that reinforce the dominant/submissive relationship between them. For instance, for dogs:

Dominant dog communication	Submissive dog communication
Making direct and intense eye contact	Looking away
Baring teeth	Mouth partly or fully closed
Growling	Whimpering
Standing tall, tail up, hackles raised, ears forward	Crouched or laid down, tail down, ears down, possibly even exposing vulnerable areas such as the belly

Each species has different dominant and submissive behaviour. In each case the different methods of communication allow animals to assert dominance or submit without having to resort to aggression or violence. The benefits of this for the group as a whole are that energy is conserved and potential injury of both animals is completely avoided.

Recognition of atypical behaviours and their cause

Atypical behaviour is behaviour that is not normally seen. Typical behaviour in one species might be atypical in another. There are a number of different atypical behaviours,

and they can be caused by different things. Observation and identification of atypical behaviour is important because it shows there is a problem which needs to be resolved.

Fear

Fear exists to help animals keep safe and it protects them in the wild. An animal that is scared will behave differently to normal. Some animals do not display fear in an obvious way but their behaviour can still reveal it.

Atypical behaviour brought on by fear can include:

- body language, such as withdrawn, submissive posture, tail between legs, crouching

- excessive panting or salivating

- displacement behaviours such as scratching, yawning etc.

- vocal sounds such as howling

- defecating (particularly noticeable for house-trained pets)

- hair or fur standing on end

Fear may be brought on by other animals

- of the same species

- of an unknown species

- of a known predator species.

Fear may be associated with humans, such as:

- strangers

- unfamiliar groups of people, such as children

- anyone that reminds the animal of past bad experiences - for instance, if they were mistreated.

Fear may also be associated with:

- loud noises

- objects

- unfamiliar places

- familiar places such as the veterinary surgery.

Fears caused by unfamiliar people may be due

to lack of contact with people when young. But this and other fears can also be due to unpleasant experiences that animals associate with the objects, places or people.

Aggression

In the wild it is in all animals' self-interest to minimise conflict because of the risk of injury and death. Both solitary and social animals find ways to avoid conflict, such as defining separate territories and agreeing on positions within social structures.

Animals who are in conflict over some resource will still try to avoid violence by behaving in a way that is meant to intimidate the other animal. One way to do this is to behave in an aggressive way. This lets the other animal know that if it came to actual violence, they would get hurt.

Aggressive behaviour in animals includes:

- making themselves look bigger, both in terms of posture, and fur or hair standing up on end (e.g. cats' tails become very large and fluffy when facing down a perceived threat)

- making plenty of noise to try and frighten the opponent (e.g. roaring in big cats, growling in dogs, chest beating in gorillas, bellowing in cows, the noise of a rattlesnake)

- other clear body language, such as bared teeth, adopting a ready-to-strike posture, or movements such as running directly at the opponent.

When there is a confrontation between different species, a threat display can come from the prospective prey, to tell the predator they should not try and attack.

If threatening behaviour does not cause one of the animals to back off then it is likely to escalate to further aggressive behaviour. This includes things like:

- chasing

- pushing, headbutting

- full-on aggression – exchanging blows, biting, scratching, or other behaviour relevant to that particular species.

Aggressive behaviour in animals in captivity may be due to any of the following:

- issues regarding territory - for instance, animals being forced to share each other's territory

- inappropriate social groups - animals that are incompatible are being forced to live together

- conflicts over food - possibly caused by the way that food is delivered e.g. there is only one feeding station

- conflicts over any other object e.g. there are not enough toys to go round

- predator and prey species can each see, hear or smell each other - this causes stress and can lead to aggressive behaviour

- protection of young animals - even the most relaxed mother will become aggressive to people or animals if there is any perceived danger to her offspring

- any perceived danger - for instance being backed into a corner

- competition for a mate during breeding time

- an animal being in pain.

Some companion animals are less socialised than others, which means that they spent little or no time with people or other animals when they were young. These animals are likely to be more aggressive with strangers and new situations than socialised animals.

Stress related behaviours (stereotypes)

Stereotypy means the repetition of a movement or action for no particular reason. In animals this would include:

- pacing up and down, or round and round

- rocking back and forth

- repeated noises

- tossing the head up and down

- moving a limb back and forth

- repeated biting or tongue movements

- chasing own tail
- excessive grooming.

Stereotypic behaviours are often linked to stress and mental well-being. They are often caused by:

- a lack of opportunity to forage for food
- poor diet
- lack of space, relative to natural behaviour in the wild
- growing up in a stressful environment.

Stereotypic behaviour is not observed in wild animals and are normally a sign that something is wrong with the captive environment.

Jargon Buster

intraspecific between animals of the same species

auditory hearing and sounds

stereotypic repeated movements for no particular reason

diurnal awake during the day, asleep at night

nocturnal asleep during the day, awake at night

crepuscular active at dawn and dusk

Quiz Questions

1 Define 'intraspecific communication'.

2 List three types of auditory communication.

3 Describe the normal social behaviour you would associate with a typical dog.

4 Define stereotypic behaviour and list some possible reasons for it.

1.2 How age, gender, environment and stress can influence behaviour

In this topics you will learn how:

- **Age differences can influence behaviour: eating, sleeping, social interactions, activity levels and movement**
- **Gender differences can influence behaviour: territorial, mating and pregnancy, social structures, parturition and egg-laying, lactation and feeding, parental investment of care**
- **Environmental factors can influence behaviour: size and design, lack of appropriate enrichment and mental stimulation, lack of companionship, lack of exercise.**

Whilst species have typical behaviour patterns, all animals are individuals and will all behave slightly differently. Certain factors may influence indviduals, such as age, gender and environment.

Age

Eating patterns

Relative to their size, young animals need to eat more to ensure they grow but their stomachs are smaller. They will eat frequently but portions will be smaller.

Older animals become less active and their nurtitional requirements decrease. They eat smaller portions and may eat less often.

Sleeping patterns

There are wide variations in the amount of sleep required by different species. However, most young mammals will sleep for longer than adults. There are likely to be many naps during the day and they may not sleep through the night when very young. Older mammals will also sleep for longer than adults.

The way in which birds sleep is similar to mammals in some ways but with some differences too. For instance, birds can sleep with only one half of their brain (and one eye open) at a time. Young birds may be more likely to sleep more than adults, because they have little else to do, but there is not a great deal of data about how much sleep birds actually need.

The concept of 'sleep' in reptiles and amphibians is different to that in mammals; reptiles may be asleep even when they look awake. You should become familiar with the behaviour that is considered normal for the species under consideration.

Social interactions

Young animals learn how to behave by interacting with other animals. They often learn important lessons for their adult life, such as hunting, through this interaction. This means that young animals will interact a great deal with each other, their parent or parents, and any other members of the extended social group. This interaction is often in the form of play - running, chasing, play-fighting and so on. this is generally the case even for solitary species.

Older animals from social species tend to lessen their interactions with other animals as they get older - particularly strangers. This is partly because of decreased activity levels and partly due to increasingly cautious behaviour.

Activity levels and movement

Whilst young animals sleep a lot, once they are awake they have a great deal of energy, and are constantly active. They will often be on the move, running and jumping a great deal.

Older animals, in contrast, become less active and their movement is more measured - less running and slower more deliberate steps.

Gender

Territorial behaviour

In the wild species often establish an area over which they roam. This allows them to access food and shelter within that area. Some species will claim this area as their own and attack animals of their own species who enter it. However most species have overlapping territories and avoid each other by visiting at different times.

The territorial instinct is strong in some animals and will be displayed in pets or domesticated animals too.

There can be differences in territorial behaviour according to gender, depending on the social behaviour of the species. For instance:

- For solitary species such as most big cats, the male's territory is likely to be larger than the female's because males seek out females to mate.

- This may not be the case for social groups. For instance, the only big cats that live in social groups are lions, where groups of males and females live together, sharing resources and defending territory together. Because of this there are no major differences between male and female lions in the size of territory.

- In general, males are often particularly aggressive to other males within their territory, as they are competitors for potential female mates. In our lion example, young male lions will leave their own pride and try to take over an existing one. This will be resisted by the males in the new pride and lead to conflict.

This kind of behaviour from males can be seen whenever they are in competition over females, including in domesticated animals - particularly when a female is ready to mate.

Mating and pregnancy

All animals have a deep instinct to pass on their genes. Animals wish to find a mate whose genes make it more likely that the offspring survive.

Female mammals are only sexually active at certain times. When this happens both female and male behaviour changes:

- females will give off visual, vocal and chemical signals that she is ready to mate

- these might include calling out, backing into males, lifting their tales to expose the genital area or other body language signs

- through these signals males will sense that females are ready to mate

- they may follow or touch females, use urine and scent to signal their availability, and become more aggressive with other males.

In a number of species this aggression turns to fights between males over claims to

the female - for example when male deer (stags) are rutting. Males may also display courtship routines. This is when animals show their prospective partner that they posses qualities that will make them the best mate. In many bird species the male is more brightly coloured than females for exactly this reason.

Once pregnant, the female's main concern is to ensure the offspring survive and her behaviour may change again as is required. This might mean, for instance, withdrawing from any further contact with males, reducing the potential for conflict to a minimum.

The male's behaviour once a female is pregnant depends on the species. For some species, the male's way to guarantee his genes are successfully passed on is to find further females to mate with. But this is not the case for all species.

Social structure

Birds and mammals have more complex social structures than reptiles, because of their reliance on one or both parents when very young. However they are rarely made up of equal numbers of males and females.

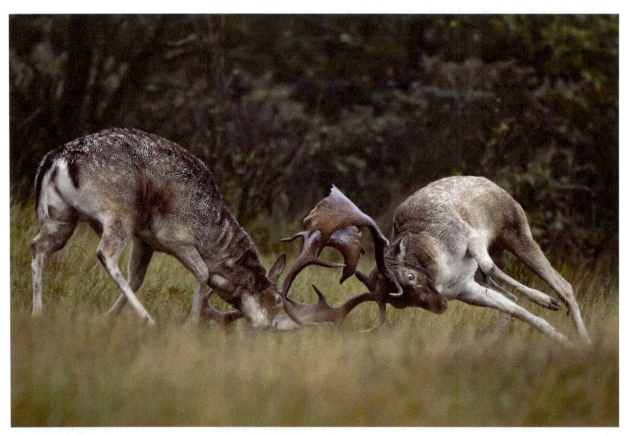

Figure 26 Rutting stags competing for females

Some examples are:

- A dominant male with a number of females and young males and females. There may be more than one adult male but if so they are lower in status than the dominant male. Examples include gorillas and wild horses.

- Groups of females and their offspring. Males are solitary and only come into contact with females for mating. Examples include pigs, feral cats.

- Similar to above, elephants form complex social group made up of females and their young. Males leave the group when they become sexually mature but may band together in small groups.

- Bird species often pair up as a mating male and female, who stay together after their parenting duties have finished. They may still be part of a larger social group too.

Apart from the paired birds, the roles of males and females, and hence their behaviour, are rarely the same in these social groups.

Parturition and egg laying

Parturition means giving birth. Mammals need a safe and quiet space to give birth in and mothers will retreat from other animals if they live in social groups. She may also try and build nests, or find a darkened solitary space, and she may stop eating.

In the case of mammals, a new mother may not wish to leave newborn animals alone for any time at all and may become aggressive if forced to do so.

Touch is an important sense for newborn animals whose other senses may not have developed at all. So new mothers may regularly lick and groom their offspring.

Birds lay eggs and and also need to find a safe spot for them, to ensure they survive. Hence they often also display nesting behaviour before laying and hatching.

Some reptiles lay eggs and some give birth to live animals like mammals. They also ensure there is a safe spot in which to give birth - but are far less maternal than mammals.

Lactation and feeding of young

One of the features that separates mammals from other animals is the ability of females to produce milk, which is called lactation. This provides offspring with nutrients from the moment of birth. This in turn means there is an important relationship between female mammals and their offspring. Evolution has led female mammals to have a natural instinct to feed and protect their newborn young. Their behaviour will change during the lactating phase in order to do this.

- They may not wish to be around other adults at all in order to keep the young safe.

- They may become very aggressive if they feel there is any threat at all to their young.

- The production of milk takes a lot of energy and, in fact, can be more difficult for animals than the pregnancy itself. So the female will need a lot of rest and will need more highly nutritious food than normal.

Young mammals will eventually move on from milk and begin to eat adult food. In the wild, this is more likely to be provided for them by their mothers, who will continue caring for them. Different species will continue this relationship for different periods of time but in some species it lasts for several years.

Birds do not produce milk but their young are also completely helpless at birth. One or both parents feed their young directly once they have hatched and so there are fewer differences between male and female behaviour. Young birds can become independent faster than many mammals and do not need looking after once they 'fly the nest'.

Parental investment of care

Different animals care for their young in different ways. There is a high cost for parents to look after their offspring – time spent looking after their young is time not spent on further reproductive activities, and finding food for the young is at the expense of their own diet. So, it is not too surprising that a great many species, such as reptiles and fish, simply do not look after their young at all. They may not even be present when the eggs hatch, leaving the young on their own from the first day.

Parental care behaviour is more complex in mammals and birds because their newborn young are often born helpless and unable to look after themselves. They need their parents to provide them with food, shelter and protection from predators. There would be an even greater cost to the parents if they didn't, as offspring would die and their genetic material would not be passed on at all.

Biparental parental care

This is when both male and female parents look after their offspring together. This is common in birds because they do not produce their own milk, and constantly finding food is very time-consuming. Sharing this task across both parents results in a greater likelihood of survival for the young birds.

Intensive parental care

It is more common in mammals for just one parent to look after the young. Because there is a high cost to parenting, if one parent can raise the young without putting the offspring at risk then the other parent does not need to be involved. This allows the other parent to find another mate.

It is normally the case that the male leaves the female to care for the young by herself. This is called maternal care and is strongly linked to the production of milk by the female. It means that an absent male has far less impact on the likelihood of survival than an absent female. Paternal care is when the male looks after the young by himself. This is much less common in animals.

Environment

The environment and surroundings of any animal in captivity can have a big impact on their behaviour.

Size and design of accommodation

Keeping any wild animal in captivity is unnatural. However, accommodation should be designed to meet the animal's needs and replicate their environment in the wild as far as possible.

The size of appropriate accommodation depends on the size of the animal and how far they travel in the wild. For instance, polar bears roam over a large territory in the wild. Their captive accommodation would therefore have to be very large.

The design of accommodation is equally important and should reflect the natural environment. This might mean lots of different levels, places to hide, different sections or zones, natural features such as trees and grass.

Livestock and some companion animals have been domesticated and do not live in the wild. But just like wild animals they have welfare needs that can only be met by ensuring they have enough space and an accommodation design that suits their species. For instance a natural roamer such as a cat is likely to display some abnormal behaviour if confined indoors.

Enrichment activities and mental stimulation

Wild animals (and the ancestors of domesticated animals) face a daily challenge to stay alive - they spend most of their time avoiding predators, finding food and mates. Each species' brain has evolved to cope with the mental stimulation provided by the complex and unpredictable wild environment. A safe captive environment however, where food is provided, removes many of the mental challenges that an animal expects to face.

As a result animals need mental stimulation to prevent them from becoming bored. This might be in the form of games or puzzles, or by encouraging foraging for food.

A lack of mental stimulation can lead to:

- inactivity
- withdrawn behaviour
- lack of interest in objects, people or other animals
- less vocal behaviour than normal

There is more in Unit 201 section 3.2 on disorders caused by lack of mental stimulation.

Companionship

Sociable animals need stimulation from their companions, so a lack of opportunities for social interaction will affect them. If such animals are starved of this when they are young, this may affect them in their adult life.

Lack of exercise

What is considered to be a normal amount of exercise depends on the species and breed. But any animal that is not doing enough exercise is likely to:

- become obsese - which can lead to serious or even fatal health problems
- exhibit destructive behaviour - for example dogs who have energy to burn.

The opportunity to exercise is related to the amount of available space.

A lack of exercise can contribute to a sense of boredom and lead to the same symptoms associated with a lack of mental stimulation.

Jargon Buster

partruition giving birth

lactation producing milk

maternal care when the mother looks after the young

paternal care when the father looks after the young

Activity

Research how age, gender, the environment and stress can affect particular aspects of behaviour in your chosen animal species.

Quiz Questions

1 Describe some of the ways in which gender affect animal behaviour.

2 How might lack of exercise affect behaviour?

3 Describe the likely changes in behaviour before and after a mammal gives birth.

1.3 Interspecific and intraspecific communication

In this topics you will learn about:

- the terms interspecific and intraspecific

- signs of communication, including human interaction: body posture, movement, vocalisation, body posture within enclosure, body posture in relation to human

- signs of relaxation, contentment, fear, aggression and stress

Animals are unable to tell us how they are feeling but they are able to communicate in other ways. It is important that you are able to understand these signs, so that you know how to behave with an animal and know what it might do next.

Animals communicate with other animals in their own species, which is known as intraspecifc communication. They also communicate with animals from different species, which is known as interspecific communication.

To remember the difference between inter- and intra, remember that intrASpecific is the SAme species

Signs of communication

Below are some general features of communication for cats and dogs. However each species has its own body language and communication behaviour so you must fully research how your selected species behaves.

Body postures

The following are key indicators for cats and dogs. However, the animal's body language as a whole must be considered to fully understand what the animal is communicating. For instance, in some breeds of dog the tail is not physically big enough to see a full range of motion. In that case other aspects of the dog's body language will help build a picture about its mood.

Ears

- ears pinned down to the head often

indicate fear in cats and dogs

- ears point up when alert or interested

Eyes

- wide eyes, showing the whites of the pupils, often demonstrates an alerted or even aggresive state

- in cats, large dilated pupils (i.e. 'saucer eyes') can be a sign of fear

- piercing, hard stares are often a sign of agitation or a direct challenge

- when the eyes look more relaxed ('soft') often the animal is too

- cats will blink slowly when relaxed

- looking away is often a sign of fear or submission

Tail

- dogs are often alert when their tail is up

- cats, however, are in a relaxed and friendly mood when their tail is up

- dogs, of course, wag their tales when relaxed - but can also wag their tails when feeling aggressive

- a wagging tail in a cat is a sign of caution, fear or aggression

- cats who are ready to attack will make their tail as big and bristly as possible

- dogs and cats tuck their tails between their legs when feeling anxious or scared

Head position

- head down can mean submission or lack of interest
- straining the head forward indicates high alert
- head on one side is a sign of interest in dogs.

Mouth

- baring teeth, unsurprisingly, is often a sign of aggression
- a dog that is 'grinning', with mouth slightly open and teeth showing a little, is excited or interested.

Facial expressions

- yawning can be a sign of stress, or a displacement activity - when an animal is caught between different urges, such as fear and curiousity about a strange object
- contorted features (i.e. screwing up the face) can indicate pain or aggression
- a snarl, unsuprisingly, indicates aggression.

Activity

Find out what body language communicates the following emotions in two animals of your choice: fear, aggression, happy/contented

Movement

The way in which an animal moves can also tell you something about its mood or intentions, when combined with posture and body language. For instance:

- an animal rushing towards another animal or person may be greeting them - but alternatively they could be preparing to attack
- an animal that runs or cowers away is frightened
- hunting animals that begin circling around another animals or person may be getting ready to attack

For cats and dogs:

- a cat making friendly gestures will walk confidently near or around people and other cats
- when in hunting mode however, cats will stalk, keeping low and stationary with small movements, making ready to pounce
- a playful dog will perform the 'play bow' - bending down on its front paws and stretching them out
- a dog that rolls over is expressing affection and wants you to pet him or her
- dogs may jump up at people as a greeting
- aggressive dogs may lunge as a warning

Activity

Find out what body movement communication signifies in your two chosen animal species.

Vocalisation

Sounds are a useful form of communication because they can send information over large distances. Vocal sounds – i.e. made with the voice – can communicate different things, such as the location of food, the call for a mate, or giving warning of predators. They can also be used to communicate threat and aggression. Vocal sounds include:

- barking
- growling,
- howling
- whimpering
- singing

Each species has their own particular vocalisation sounds.

Activity

Research some common vocalisations for your two chosen animal species.

Body position within enclosure

Animals who are scared will make sure they can see all potential threats, make their body small and have an escape route. Animals with a defensive body posture positioned at the back of the enclosure, away from the entrance or in any hidden areas, may be anxious or afraid. Fearful animals can quickly turn aggressive.

Animals who have a relaxed pose lying nearer in full view or near the entrance are likely to be approachable.

Animals stalking or pacing around, running at the entrance, or standing still and staring hard are likely to be agitated or aggressive.

If an animal from a sociable species is keeping well away from other animals in the enclosure then there may be a problem with the social group. For instance there may be a clash between dominant males. Alternatively the animal might be ill.

In all cases however the mood of the animal based on body position can only be assessed along with their body language.

Body position in relation to human

The position of an animal must be assessed along with its posture and any other signs it is giving. However, an animal that is slowly approaching, with a curious or interested posture, is unlikely to be a threat as long as there are no sudden movements or anything else to scare it.

A familiar animal approaching more quickly, with a friendly or excited demeanour, is likely to be giving a greeting. However an unfamiliar animal should be treated with more caution as excitement can quickly turn to more aggressive actions.

An animal rushing towards a human at speed may pose a threat. An animal that darts towards a person before retreating is giving a warning to keep away. An animal that is

backing away is afraid - but may lash out in defensive aggression.

Any animal that is backed into a corner may feel under threat, even if that is far from the intention of the person backing them in. This may cause them to lash out. Animals should always be given an escape route to prevent this.

Activity

Find out what body positions relative to humans are common in your two chosen animal species.

Signs of relaxation and contentment, fear, aggression and stress

As discussed, animals communicate how they are feeling in a number of ways, including their body language and facial expressions. However, whilst there are some general trends, each animal species has its own specific communication methods.

For your chosen species you will need to understand the signs that communicate the following moods:

- contentment
- fear
- aggression
- stress.

As an example, some visual signs of four moods are given in figures 24 and 25 for cats and dogs.

Jargon Buster
intraspecific between the same species

interspecific between different species

Quiz Questions

1 How might a cat communicate fear through its a) eyes, b) tail, c) vocalisations.

2 Describe how your chosen species might communicate aggression.

3 It is feeding time and a rescue dog you have never met is pacing back and forth at the front of their cage, looking directly at you. What action should you take?

LO2 Monitor and record behaviour in animals

2.1 Carry out behaviour observations

2.2 Record and report on behaviour observations

> **In these next two topics you will learn about:**
>
> - **the reasons for and methods of observation: the effect of observer position, duration and frequency of observation, ethograms, sampling methods, observation of individuals and groups**
>
> - **recording and reporting observations: what to record, format, recording findings legibly, written reports, oral reports**

We have discussed how an animal's actions can communicate how they are feeling at that particular moment. For this to be useful, people working with animals routinely observe them and record their findings. There are a few different reasons why observations are made:

- monitoring general health and well-being of individuals

- monitoring animals with known or suspected health conditions, or with special requirements (for instance, pregnant animals)

- to understand the behaviour of particular individuals or groups of interest

- to understand behaviour as part of wider research and study of the animal species or breed.

Observations allow carers to build a picture of patterns of behaviour, which helps them understand all of their needs and also spot any potential problems at the earliest stage.

Some thought has to be given to the method of observation, its frequency and how to record it.

Obtrusive and unobtrusive position of observer

Observations can take place in person. This is simple to set up. However there are a few disadvantages:

- The presence of the observer may afffect the behaviour of the animal. If this happens then the observations will not monitor the animal's natural behaviour. Whether this is a problem or not depends on the aim of the observation. It also depends on the animal itself, as some will be used to humans and not behave differently in front of them.

- In-person observations are less suitable for long timeframes, If 24 hour observations are required, this would take a team of people with considerable commitment and patience.

- In-person observations are less suitable for brief or irregular encounters. Spending hours and hours waiting for an animal to appear may not always be the best use of time.

To prevent the observer having an impact on behaviour, hides can be used. These allow an observer to remain hidden from the animal. As many animals have an excellent sense

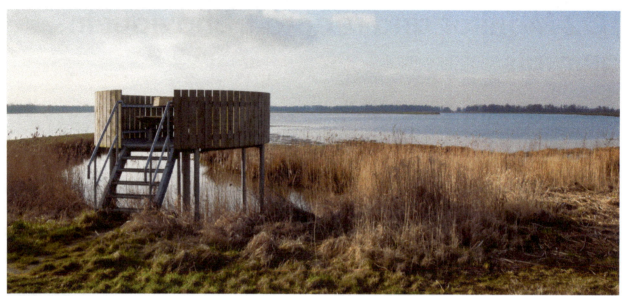

Figure 27 A hide used for observing birds

of smell, observers should also aim to be downwind when they want to remain hidden.

An alternative to in-person observation is to use a video camera instead. The advantages of a video camera are:

- its presence will not affect animal behaviour

- it can be used for remote monitoring, with footage broadcast to a different site

- special cameras can be equipped with night-vision to observe nocturnal animas

- cameras can be combined with motion sensors so that only useful footage is captured.

There are some disadvantages too:

- basic cameras cannot move or zoom - so if something takes place just out of shot then the moment is missed

- someone still has to either watch the broadcast live, or view the recorded footage

- there is the possibility of a technical failure

- more expensive to set up and run.

You can see an example of a video camera set up to record animal behaviour in this YouTube footage:

https://tinyurl.com/dx4vvt3

Duration and frequency of observation

Duration means how long the observation is for and frequency means how often the observation is. Both depend on the aim of the observation.

- For instance, in an animal welfare shelter the aim would be to monitor general and specific health conditions and well-being. So observations would be at least once per day, and would probably focus on key moments of the day, such as feeding times, as eating problems can be an indicator of many different conditions. These observations would carry on all through the year.

- Another observation might aim to more clearly understand mating behaviour of particular species within a bird sanctuary. In which case each observation might be longer but spread out over daylight hours. The observations would only be for a limited amount of time - for instance, one month - as the breeding season then comes to an end.

The important thing is that duration and frequency choices have been thought out carefully in advance rather than arrived at by accident when performing the observation; and thought is given as to why the duration and frequency might be appropriate, given the aims of the observation.

Behaviour	Behaviour code	Description
Eating	E	Animal is eating food
Drinking	D	Animal is drinking water
Sleeping	S	Animal is fully asleep, eyes closed.
Resting	R	Animal is laid down, not moving but eyes are open and is not asleep
Vocalisation - barking	VB	Animal is barking
Vocalisation - whimpering	VW	Animal is making a high-pitch whimpering sound

Figure 28 An ethogram

Ethograms

An ethogram (figure 28) is a list of animal behaviour split into different categories and sub-categories. Once the ethogram categories have been created then observations record the amount of time that the animal displays each category of behaviour.

The aim of an ethogram is to allow observers to record behaviour objectively and accurately, so that comparisons over time, and with different animals, are fair. This means that the ethogram behaviours should be written objectively. The idea is that you just record precisely what the animal(s) is doing - not **why** you think it is behaving that way. This is because assumptions about the reasons for an animal's behaviour may be wrong.

You can create your own ethogram by writing down the different behaviour that you expect to see in an animal you observe. Ethogram categories can be very simple, or very complex with many different behaviours listed. The more complicated the ethogram the more involved the observation itself.

Sampling methods

Observing animals is a scientific process. This means we need to be sure we are not accidentally recording data that is somehow biased. A potential problem with observations is that they miss certain behaviours but emphasise others. This might be because it focuses on only one animal, or only when an animal is doing something 'interesting'. This would be misleading.

Sampling is a way to minimise these problems. It can take a few different forms such as:

- recording an animal or group continuously for a set amount of time, and at the same times, each day - this is called focal sampling

- only recording an animal or group at set intervals for a certain duration, for instance every minute for twenty minutes - this is called instantaneous scan sampling

- only recording interesting or important behaviour is called ad lib sampling - whilst it can be misleading it is sometimes useful to record unusual behaviour.

Sampling methods are designed to ensure that an animal's real behaviour is captured. So the exact details of the sample - how often, how many times a day, over how many days and so on, will depend on the aim of the observation in the first place.

Observation of individuals and groups

The choice of observing individuals or groups depends on the aim of the observation. If welfare is being tracked then part of that observation will need to focus on each individual. If dynamics at feeding time is under investigation then groups will need to be studied.

Observing a group has different challenges from observing an individual and may require a different ethogram and sampling method.

Record and report on behaviour observations

For observations to be useful they should be clearly recorded, so that other people can view and understand them at a later date.

What to record

Some key information needs to be recorded accurately and consistently in each observation:

- animal identified
- date and time
- duration of observation
- behaviours seen - as categorised by an ethogram if using one

Format of recording behaviour

Behaviour can be recorded in the following ways:

- using pen and blank paper
- using printed templates that are filled in
- descriptions should be brief and factual rather than descriptive
- drawings can also help communicate postures and physical behaviour - they do not have to be works of art, simple stick drawings can be very useful
- if using an ethogram, graphical methods could be used to communicate different duration of each behaviour
- computer progams or smartphone apps can be used instead of pen and paper.

Record all findings legibly

It is important that all handwritten notes are easy to read. If any mistakes are made cross out with one or two straight lines and carry on.

Written reports on records

Reports are documents that summarise recorded data and draw conclusions. The exact style of a written report depends on its purpose but in all cases it should be professional, with good spelling and grammar. If handwritten then it should also be easy to read for someone else.

More formal reports might be longer and written using a word-processor. More frequent reports (i.e. weekly findings in a cattery) may be shorter.

Oral reports

In some settings it may be normal to report your observations and findings to someone in person such as:

- your supervisor
- your employer
- any other person in charge

Even if this is not the case, you will need to report anything you have observed that requires immediate attention, for instance a fight that has left one animal injured, a possible health hazard that was spotted in an enclosure, and so on.

Jargon Buster

biased where the design of an experiment affects the results

ethogram a list of animal behaviour, split into categories; useful when sampling

focal sampling sampling for the same amount of time, at the same time of day

instantaneous scan sampling recording for sets amount of time over a set time interval

ad lib sampling only recording apparently important or unusual behaviour

---

Quiz Questions

1 What is an 'ethogram' used for?

2 List two sampling methods and describe the main features of each.

3 Describe the advantages and disadvantages of unobtrusive observations.

4 How might observations be recorded?

LO3 Handle and restrain animals safely

3.1 Assess and approach animals

In this topic you will learn about:

- **Assessing animals before approaching them.**

Well before handling, an animal's mood, temperament and behaviour should be assessed. As discussed in the previous section, animals' body language and other signals communicates how it is feeling and what it might do next. Questions to be asked include:

- is the animal in pain?
- are there any signs of fear?
- are there any signs of aggression?
- are there any other special circumstances to consider - such as the presence of other animals that might cause the mood to change quickly?

The animals' signals should be carefully considered as a whole, with regard to the species in question, before taking any further action.

If it is considered safe then the next stage is to approach. Animals will also assess you as you approach, so you need to ensure that they do not see you as a threat. This can be done by

- Approaching animals slowly, calmly but confidently.
- Speaking to the animal in a reassuring manner, keeping your voice low.
- Using slow and smooth movements and never making sudden gestures.
- Adopting appropriate body posture and body language.
- Always allowing an escape route for the animal - do not back them into a corner.

Appropriate body language will be different for different species. For instance, dogs will think that approaching from the front, stretching out a hand and looking directly into their eyes is a challenge or even a threat. Avoiding direct eye contact and turning slightly to the side is a much better approach.

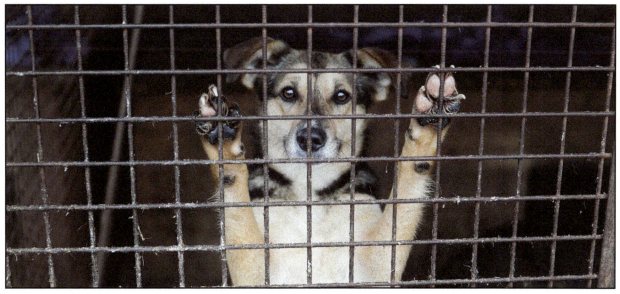

Figure 29 This dog would need to be carefully assessed before approaching

3.2 Use correct handling and equipment and techniques for animals

In this topic you will learn about:

• Selecting the appropriate Personal Protective Equipment (PPE) when handling animals

• Selecting the handling equipment appropriate for the species

• The handling technique needs to be appropriate for selected scenarios: exercising and heath checks

PPE

Personal Protective Equipment (PPE) should be worn to keep safe from hazards. Hazards include the risk of bites and scratches, the risk of disease, or the risk of passing disease on to other animals.

Typical PPE for animal handlers includes:

• Gloves and gauntlets: hands are an obvious target for any animal that is not happy at being handled, so gloves and gauntlets are used to keep the hands and arms covered. If they are thick enough they can protect from the bites and scratches of smaller animals.

• Eye protection: goggles and visors keep the eyes safe from any substance that might come into contact with them. They are also a line of defence against larger animals who might be able to reach the face with their claws.

• Face masks: these protect the mouth from splashes of any animal substances. Whilst they can help reduce airborne transmission of germs they do not provide full protection. So if an animal has a zoonotic disease that is spread through the air, different PPE (such as breathing apparatus) would be needed instead.

• Protective clothing: hard-wearing clothes should cover all skin (i.e. long sleeves and long trousers). Disposable coverings such as aprons, gowns and covering for shoes might also be required to prevent the spread of disease.

• Sturdy closed shoes: no sandals or open-toed shoes to ensure no skin is exposed.

• Clothes should not be loose, and no scarves, bracelets, earrings or jewellery of any kind should be worn. This is to prevent animals being able to catch hold of any items.

Handling equipment

Different equipment is needed for handling different species. You must select the best equipment for the species, and animal, in question. Typical handling equipment includes:

• Collars and leads: these provide a way to prevent animals from escaping. Standard collars may not be suitable for small dogs, those with narrow necks or those with breathing issues (e.g. pugs).

• Crush cages: these are used to treat wild animals or animals that are likely to scratch or bite. A movable wall can gently push the animal against one side of the cage where they can be treated - for instance with an injection. Crush bags perform a similar function but the body and limbs are enlosed in a bag instead.

• Muzzles for cats and dogs: these hold the mouth in place and prevent bites.

• Graspers and nooses: these are made up of metal or plastic poles with a noose or grasper at the end. With the noose or grasper secured carefully around the animal's neck, these prevent animals approaching the handler. They are vital for handling larger or very aggressive animals.

• towels and blankets: these can be used to

wrap smaller animals and then hold them in place to ensure they cannot move. They can be used to stop animals running away and to prevent any scratching.

- Head collar and harnesses: harnesses fit over the shoulders and chest, and are used to provide more control and comfort for larger, stronger animals.

Handling techniques for selected scenarios

Two common reasons for handling an animal are exercise and health checks.

Exercising

Animals that need exercise often require handling to fit equipment as well as for the exercise itself. Different animals require different equipment but the key points are:

- ensure the animal is safe to approach first
- fit any equipment safely - making sure, for instance, that collars are not too tight or too loose
- make sure that any restraints are not causing any discomfort or pain
- only use the equipment for its intended purpose
- for any animal nervous of humans, minimise the time spent touching the animal directly

Health check

Animals need handling during any health check or procedure. These events can be quite frightening for animals because:

- they often take place in an unfamiliar location, e.g. a veterinary surgery, with unusual smells, sounds and sights

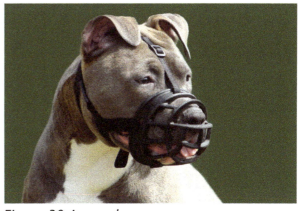

Figure 30 A muzzle

- the animal is likely to have been transported there, which they may have found traumatic
- the presence of other animals and strangers may be unsettling
- some parts of the check-up may be uncomfortable.

Frightened animals are more likely to behave unpredictably or aggressively, so great care needs to be taken when working with them. They should always be kept in clear sight - never have a back turned to them when out of a cage.

They may need to be kept in cages before and after the check up, to prevent them running away, and aggressive animals may even need to be kept in a cage during treatment.

Consideration should be given to the effect other animals might have. Species that are likely to cause each other great stress should be kept far apart.

To minimise the stress of the situation, animals should be handled as little as possible.

Jargon Buster
gauntlet a thick and long glove

Quiz Questions

1 Why might PPE be used when handling animals?

2 Outline the correct way to approach a dog.

3 Explain the purpose of a crush cage.

4 List two items of equipment that might required when handling animals.

3.3 Situations that would require handling with extreme care

In this topic you will learn about situations that would require handling of animals with extreme care or alternative equipment, the limitations of own experience and skills when handling animals, when to seek help from more experienced colleagues, in the following scenarios:

- Newly arrived at rehab or veterinary centre

- Late pregnancy

- During birth (unless vital due to birthing problems)

- During early lactation

- Directly following surgery

- Seriously ill

- No supervisor or assistant present if procedure requires help

- Animal is showing signs of aggression

Animal handling covers a wide variety of animals, species and possible scenarios. There are certain situations that require particular care and attention.

In all situations, but particularly in these cases, anyone handling an animal must ask themselves:

- do I have the skills and experience to deal with this situation?

- when would be a sensible time to ask someone more experienced for help?

It is far more desirable to anticipate a difficult situation and ask for help or advice in advance, rather than waiting for a situation to unfold.

Newly arrived at rehab or veterinary centre

New arrivals are likely to be afraid of their new surroundings. This includes the environment, the people and the other animals. This would result in more nervous behaviour than normal, or possibly signs of aggression.

They might require more gentle coaxing than

normal, and animals may need to be given more time to get used to their surroundings.

Late pregnancy

In the later stages of pregnancy an animal may be in discomfort. They may also have a very natural desire to be alone. Any handling should therefore be kept to a minimum during this stage and consideration given to the physical condition of the animal.

During birth

Birth should be allowed to happen naturally without any interference. Only if there are medical problems should there be any interaction with the animal. In this case, however, only suitably qualified persons should attempt to help. If you have not had any training and you suspect there is a problem then you should find help as soon as possible. Ideally an experienced person would be available before the animal gives birth.

During early lactation

Many young animals during the lactation

(milking) phase are very vulnerable and rely on their mothers for protection. There are many dangers for the young in the wild and so new mothers are very protective. Contact with young animals during this phase can lead to serious aggression from the mother and should therefore be minimised as far as possible.

In some species handling the young animals can lead to them being rejected by the mother - in such species it is critical that they are not handled unless there is a clear medical reason.

Directly following surgery

After surgery animals will probably be in some pain, have restricted movement and in need of rest. Again, they may behave unexpectedly as a result and should be assessed very carefully before approaching. Handling should be minimised and the animal allowed to rest.

Seriously ill

A seriously ill animal must be assessed quickly to see whether it requires immediate help, to prevent loss of life or serious injury. First aid can be given if necessary but only if trained in the basic procedures.

The aims of first aid are covered in Unit 201 section 4.

Any animal that is ill or has been injured is likely to be scared and might be in pain. They are far more likely to act aggressively, even if this is completely out of character. Approaching any seriously ill animal must only be done with the greatest of care, and any equipment that can prevent biting or scratching should be used as a precaution - assuming it will not further injure the animal.

For animals who are seriously ill but do not require first aid or emergency treatment, the approach is the same as that following surgery. Try to keep them comfortable and handle them as little as possible.

No supervisor or assistant present if procedure requires help

If a handling procedure requires help, but no one is available to assist, then the animal should not be handled - you must wait until someone is available.

Animal is showing signs of aggression

Any animal that needs to be handled but is showing signs of aggression will require some special techniques and/or equipment. There should be someone present who has experience of dealing with aggressive animals - ideally with experience of the species in question. If you do not have this experience then you must not approach the animal. For this reason, it is very important that an animal is carefully assessed for aggressive behaviour before approaching.

If an animal is showing signs of aggression whilst still in a cage then attempts should be made to calm it down by lowering the light levels and removing other animals.

Quiz Questions

1 Explain why might special handling procedures be put in place for a pregnant cat in a shelter,

2 Describe how you would handle a horse who had recently had surgery on her hoof.

Unit 229 Working in the animal care industry

LO1 Know the structure of the animal care industry

1.1 Job roles

In this topic you will learn about duties of different roles in the animal care industry:

• Animal care assistant

• Trainee animal care worker

• Trainee pet store assistant

• Trainee kennel or cattery worker

There are a number of different roles within the animal care industry, each with different duties.

Animal care assistant

An animal care assistant is an entry-level position, which could be based at a rescue centre, animal centre or wildlife park. They would assist an animal care worker. Typical duties include:

• cleaning and grooming animals

• feeding animals

• exercising, socialising and training animals.

Trainee animal care worker

An animal care worker could be based in a rescue centre, animal centre or wildlife park. A trainee will build on their previous experience and knowledge gained from a qualification such as this one, whilst performing a range of directed tasks. Typical duties include:

• monitoring animals' health

• keeping accommodation clean

• cleaning animals

• helping to prepare food and help with feeding animals

• exercising animals

• maintaining living areas

• working with distressed, ill or injured animals.

Trainee pet store assistant

Working in a pet shop involves looking after the animal residents in a retail environment. This means there will be lots of interaction with the general public, and animals regularly arriving and leaving. Typical duties include:

• feeding animals

• cleaning out cages and living areas

• cleaning and grooming animals

• exercising animals

• selling products and equipment associated with pets

• advising customers who are looking for pets

- keeping the premises clean and tidy

- dealing with deliveries

- helping to manage stock

- working with computer systems.

Trainee kennel or cattery worker

This role is similar to an animal care worker but is based specifically in a kennel or cattery. Typical duties include:

- monitoring animals' health

- keeping accommodation clean

- cleaning and grooming animals

- helping to prepare food and help with feeding animals

- exercising animals and in the case of dogs, taking them for walks

- maintaining living areas and exercise grounds

- dealing with the general public, either in person or on the telephone.

Quiz Questions

1 Describe the main responsibilities of a trainee animal care worker.

1.2 Industry associations

- In this topic you will learn about the following animal industry associations:

- Pet Industry Federation (PIF)

- Royal Society for the Prevention of Cruelty to Animals (RSPCA)

- Blue Cross

- Guide Dogs for the Blind

- British and Irish Association of Zoos and Aquariums (BIAZA)

- British Veterinary Association (BVA)

- Royal College of Veterinary Surgeons

(RCVS)

- Department of Environment, Food and Rural Affairs (Defra)

- The Kennel Club

- Cats Protection

- People's Dispensary for Sick Animals (PDSA)

- British Veterinary Nursing Association (BVNA)

Industry associations are organisations that represent particular groups within the animal industry. Their precise roles are discussed as follows.

Pet Industry Federation (PIF)

This organisation represents the pet industry in the UK. This includes retailers (i.e. shops), companies that make pet equipment, kennels, catteries, dog walkers, pet sitters and grooming parlours.

It provides a number of services for members and ensures that the pet industry in the UK is represented.

Royal Society for the Prevention of Cruelty to Animals (RSPCA)

This is an animal welfare charity. They work to prevent cruelty, prevent suffering and promote kindness and compassion to all animals.

They rescue animals in danger and prosecute those who break the UK's animal welfare laws. They also campaign for changes to laws where necessary, run rescue centres, and raise awareness of animal welfare issues through education.

Blue Cross

This animal welfare charity helps rehome and adopt unwanted pets, provides veterinary services through animal hospitals, and runs education campaigns on animal welfare issues.

Guide Dogs for the Blind

This charity provides guide dogs to partially-sighted and blind people in the UK. They breed and train the dogs, which is a complex, demanding and expensive task. They also campaign on behalf of issues affecting blind and partially-sighted people.

British and Irish Association of Zoos and Aquariums (BIAZA)

This is the professional body that represents zoos and aquariums in the UK and Ireland. Their work includes the promotion of conservation programmes in the wild, supporting research, and helping members deliver the best standards of animal welfare. They also deliver campaigns to raise awareness of conservation issues with the public.

British Veterinary Association (BVA)

This membership organisation represents veterinary surgeons in the UK. They provide members with training and educational material to help keep them up to date, research journals, careers advice and job vacancies, as well as other benefits.

The BVA also campaigns on behalf of vets and represents them when discussing with issues with the government.

Royal College of Veterinary Surgeons (RCVS)

A veterinary surgeon is a restricted job title - the only people who can call themselves veterinary surgeons have to be suitably qualified. The same is true of veterinary nurses. The RCVS are responsible for keeping a register of all qualified veterinary surgeons and veterinary nurses who are allowed to work in the UK. They also uphold the standards to which vets have to uphold, and regulate the professional conduct of vets.

The RCVS also works to research veterinary science and promote education among its members.

Department of Environment, Food and Rural Affairs (Defra)

Defra is a government department that is responsible in England for the food, farming and fisheries industries, overseeing the protection of the natural environment, and for the rural economy.

They oversee all laws relating to the welfare and treatment of animals.

The Kennel Club

This membership organisation is devoted to the promotion of health, welfare and training in dogs. They run a register for breeders, run dog training programmes, run Crufts (see next page), and educate and advise dog owners on welfare and training issues. They also support research into diseases which affect dogs. Members are entitled to a range of other benefits too.

Cats Protection

This charity is dedicated to the welfare of cats in the UK. They find new homes for unwanted pets, encourage the neutering of cats, and provide education and information so that people can better understand cats' needs and how to care for them. They also provide help for those suffering with grief from the loss of a pet, and campaign on issues affecting cats and cat ownership.

People's Dispensary for Sick Animals (PDSA)

This charity aims to prevent pet animal illness and suffering by providing free or low-cost veterinary help for pets whose owners cannot afford it. They run a number of animal hospitals in the UK for this purpose. They also campaign on behalf of issues affecting pet animals and their owners.

British Veterinary Nursing Association (BVNA)

This is a membership body for veterinary nurses. It provides training, education, research, events and legal advice for all veterinary nurse members in the UK. It represents veterinary nurses and their interests, and promotes the profession with government and other relevant organisations.

Quiz Questions

1 List three animal industry associations.

2 Describe the role that Defra plays.

3 Name the organisations that are specifically aimed at people working in veterinary surgeries.

1.3 Industry events

In this topic you will learn about the following animal industry events:

- Pet and Aquatic Trade Show (PATS)
- Crufts
- British Dog Grooming Championship
- K9 Expo
- The National/British Pet Show
- The London Vet Show
- BSAVA Congress

Pet and Aquatic Trade Show (PATS)

Purpose: A trade show for the pet and aquatic industries. It provides an opportunity for businesses, manufacturers and retailers to display their products and make connections with prospective customers.

Activities: Seminars and dog grooming demonstrations.

Key dates: February and September each year.

Crufts

Purpose: This event is run by the Kennel Club and is a celebration of dogs. It is the largest of its kind in the world. The famous part of the event is the dog show, covering numerous different categories and events. But there is also a trade exhibition for manufacturers and retailers of dog-related products and services.

Activities: A prestigious dog conformation show - that is, where animals are judged as to how closely they conform to the standards of their breed. This means that the dogs are not being compared directly to each other.

Other activities include dog agility competitions, obedience competitions, heelwork to music competitions, and flyball - a team sport for dogs!

Key dates: March each year.

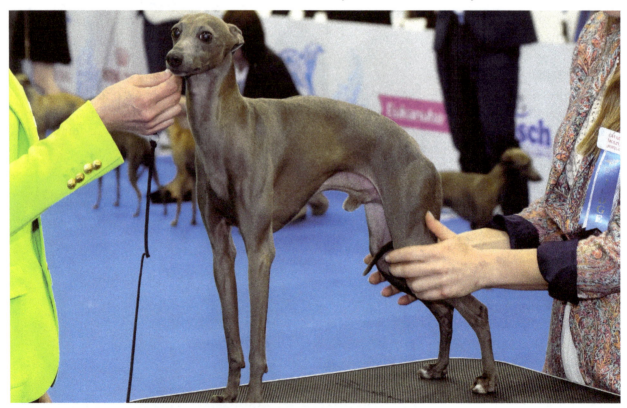

Figure 31 A dog being examined at a dog conformation show

British Dog Grooming Championship

Purpose: A competition for professional dog groomers, organised by the Pet Industry Federation.

Activities: There are various classes of competitor (e.g. Beginner, Advanced) and breed of dog. Competitors will then groom dogs in front of a judging panel.

Key dates: April each year.

K9 Expo

Purpose: To promote dog grooming skills in Northern Ireland.

Activities: Dog grooming competition.

Key dates: Check website.

The National/British Pet Show

Purpose: Aimed at animal lovers, this show is a chance for the general public to meet animals, listen to educational talks from experts and discover more about owning and looking after pets.

Activities: 'Meet the animals', talks from experts and speciality breeders, educational sessions about owning different animals, and a chance to meet rescued animals.

Key dates: October/November each year.

The London Vet Show

Purpose: Information and education show aimed at the UK and international veterinary professionals.

Activities: Conference programme containing expert speakers covering all aspects of veterinary science.

Trade exhibition, to connect manufacturers and retailers with vets and veterinary professionals.

Key dates: November each year.

BSAVA Congress

Purpose: Run by the British Small Animal Veterinary Association, this event is aimed at veterinary professionals who specialise in companion animals.

Activities: Conference and education programme with expert speakers discussing issues relevant to small animals.

Exhibition to connect manufacturers and retailers with veterinary professionals.

Key dates: Spring each year.

> **Jargon Buster**
> conformation show a judging competition where animals' characteristics are compared to the best possible examples from their breed

Quiz Questions

1 Outline the main activities that take place at Crufts.

2 List the possible attendees of the Pet and Aquatic Trade Show.

LO2 Know employment rights and responsibilities

2.1 Employment rights

2.2 Employee responsibilities

In these topics you will learn about the employment rights of employees:

- **Safe working environment**
- **Training**
- **Rest periods**
- **Holidays**

- **Minimum wage**
- **Living wage**
- **Contract of payment**

You will also learn about the responsibilities of employees:

- **Punctuality**
- **Safety of others**

- **Maintain the working environment**

Employees have a number of rights which are protected in law. It is important that you understand your rights as an employee.

NOTE: The following rights apply to employees or workers, not self-employed people. Very rarely, some employers may claim their staff are self-employed, to deny them these rights. If you are in any doubt about your employment status (i.e. a worker, an employee or self-employed) you should seek some professional advice.

Safe working environment

Employers have a responsibility to provide a safe working environment for their employees. In Unit 202 Section 3.3 we discussed the Health and Safety at Work Act (1974) in relation to cleaning animal accommodation. This law applies to all aspects of the working environment and employers can be prosecuted if they are in breach of the Act (i.e. they have broken the law).

Note that under the Act employees also have responsibilities too.

Training

An employee has the right to ask their employer for time off in order to undertake training or study. The important points are:

- The legal requirement only applies to organisations with over 250 employees. (Smaller organisations may still be open to the idea if they can see that it will benefit their business).

- The training or study must be relevant and likely to help the employee in their job.

- The employer does not have to pay for the training or study.

- The employee must have worked for the employer for at least 26 weeks before the request.

The employer has to give serious consideration to the request but they can refuse if the absence meant they could not run their business properly, if it was likely to cost the business money, or if the training was not related to the employer's job.

Rest periods

If you are over 16 but under 18 you are entitled to a minimum of:

- a 30 minute rest if you work 4.5 hours in one day

- 12 hours of rest between working days

- 2 days off per week.

Note that at this age you are not normally allowed to work more than 8 hours a day or 40 hours per week. You are also not allowed to work overnight between 10pm - 6am (or 11pm - 7am) the following day.

If you are over 18 and work more than 6 hours in a day you are entitled to a minimum of:

- a 20 minute break at some point during that 6 hours

- 11 hours of rest between working days

- 1 day off every week (or 2 days off every fortnight).

Holidays

Full-time employees are entitled to a minimum of 5.6 weeks (or 28 days) of paid holiday per year. This means that you are still paid your normal wage even when you are not at work.

There are 8 bank holidays in England and Wales, so employers often choose to use the bank holidays as part of the allowance. This means you would get 20 days (four weeks) of holiday plus another 8 days on bank holidays.

There is no exact definition but full-time work is often classed as working 35 hours or more per week (or 5 days per week for 7 hours per day).

Part-time workers are entitled to the same benefits but in proportion to their hours worked (which is known as 'pro rata'). So, for instance, if someone worked 17.5 hours per week (which is half of the full-time 35 hours), then they would be entitled to 14 days (2.8 weeks) paid holiday per year. This would give them the same amount of time off because they only need to take 2.5 days to have a whole week off.

National Minimum Wage and National Living Wage

There is a minimum wage per hour, set out in law, that employers must pay their employees. The exact details of the minimum wage often changes each April. The rates are set out in bands according to age and there is also a special rate for apprentices.

The current bands are:

- Apprentices

- Under 18

- 18-20

- 21-24

- 25 and over

These minimum rates tend to increase with each age band, with people aged 25 and over having the highest minimum wage. (For historical reasons, the minimum wage for people aged 25 and over is referred to as the National Living Wage.)

> **Activity**
>
> Find out what the current National Minimum Wage and National Living Wage rates are. Which rate applies to you?

Contract of payment

An employer must give you a written statement, containing certain terms and conditions of your employment, within two months of starting work. However even before anything is in writing, a contract still exists between you and your employer as soon as you begin working for them.

There are certain things that a contract must cover. Perhaps the most important is that you have a right to be paid for the work that you do, the times of the day that you are expected to work, the total hours of work each week or month, and the wages for that work.

A contract can contain lots of different agreements between you and your employer but it cannot override any rights you have in law. For instance, it could not state that you were to be paid less than the minimum wage.

Employee responsibilities

Whilst employers have certain legal responsibilities as discussed, employees also have responsibilities.

Punctuality

The contract of employment will state the hours that an employee is expected to work and be paid for. It may also state the start and end time of the working day, or this may be agreed verbally with the employer. In either case the employee must be at their workplace and ready to begin work at the start of their contracted hours. This is referred to as being punctual or on time.

- If it takes some time to get ready before work can begin - for instance, because the employee needs to put on special clothes or a uniform - then the employee must factor this in and arrive earlier.

- If it is likely that there will be delays on the journey to work (for instance caused by traffic) then the employee must factor this in and set off to work earlier.

Being punctual means that the employee is fulfilling their side of the employment contract. But perhaps even more importantly it also shows that the employee is acting professionally and is taking their job seriously.

Safety of others

We have already touched upon the Health and Safety at Work Act (1974). In that Act there are legal requirements for the employee to give due care to the health and safety of themselves and others in the working environment. This includes helping and co-operating with their employer as they also act to provide a safe working environment.

Employee responsibilities here would include:

- Reporting any potentially dangerous situations in the working environment, so that the employer can prevent anyone being injured - for instance, spillages that could result in slips, broken glass that could cause cuts, any fire hazard etc.

- Not interfering with measures put in place by the employer with regard to health and safety - for instance, tampering or moving 'danger' signs, leaving fire doors propped open, altering safety mechanisms on equipment, or approaching animals that have been instructed to be left alone.

- Paying full and proper attention to any training that the employee receives and putting the training into action on a day-to-day basis - for instance, after being given training on lifting objects in a safe and correct manner, the employee must not then continue to lift heavy objects by themselves back in the workplace.

- Taking full notice of fire drills and following all directions associated with them.

Maintain the working environment

Whist employees have a responsibility to report any problems, dangers or hazards, employees also have a responsibility to keep the workplace clean and safe to prevent hazards in the first place. This means applying the principles of cleaning and maintenance routines covered in Unit 202 to all aspects of the work environment. You can keep on top of any problems and prevent hazards by:

- replacing or reporting worn-out items

- packing items of equipment away safely when not in use

- never leaving equipment lying around, particularly in dangerous areas such as stairs, or in kitchens where people may be carrying hot water or knives

- ensuring germs cannot gather and spread disease by keeping all areas clean

Jargon Buster
pro rata a latin term that means 'in proportion' - so in the context of pay and holidays it means in proportion to a full-time employee

LO3 Understand the organisation of business

3.1 Business structures

3.2 Organisational policies

3.3 Promotion of the organisation

In these topics you will learn about the organisation of business:

- **Different types of business: Sole trader, Limited company, Partnership, Franchise, Chain**

- **Content of different types of organisation policies: Health and safety, Complaints, Dress code, Use of social media, Attendance, Store presentation, Professional standards**

- **Suitability of types of organisation promotion: Displays, Posters, Leaflets, Websites, Social media, Events**

- **Implications of promotion using social media: Use of personal social media, Negative social media comments, e-safety**

Business structures

A business can be set up in a number of different ways. Each different business structure listed has a different legal definition and has different legal requirements regarding the way they declare profits and pay tax.

Sole trader

This is the simplest business structure. As the name suggests it is set up by one person who takes full responsibility for all aspects of running the business. This person is self-employed. Key points about a sole trader are:

- It is simple and easy to set up a sole trader business - you simply choose a name to trade under and register for tax (see below).

- Any profits made by the business belong to the sole trader themselves.

- The sole trader has to complete a self-assessment tax return to the government (the tax-collecting department called HMRC) each year, declaring their profits.

- The business and the individual are the same in the eyes of the law. This means that if the business ran up debts that it could not pay, the sole trader's personal items of value (called assets) could be used to pay those debts - for instance, their house. The technical term for this is that the sole trader has unlimited liability.

Limited company

A limited company is a more formal business structure that aims to make a profit. The main difference between it and a sole trader is that a limited company is, in legal terms, separate from the person or people who set it up.

To set up a limited company one or more shareholders registers the company name with a body called Companies House. The shareholder(s) appoint one or more directors to run the company. The shareholders initially invest some money in the new company which is recorded as shares in the company. The shares can be worth any amount. If one person sets up a new limited company they can set it up with one share worth only £1!

The important points about limited companies are:

- They are more complicated to set up as they have to be registered with Companies House, details about directors and shareholders have to be recorded, and there is a requirement to keep various records.

- A shareholder can also be a director of the company but does not have to be. This means that the owners of the company can be separate from the people running the company.

- The profits made by the limited company belong to the limited company - they do

not belong to the owner/shareholder or the director. Instead, shareholders and directors can be paid by the company (in different ways).

- The company is required to file its accounts every year and pay tax on any profits it makes.

- The financial risk of the shareholders is limited to how much money they have invested as shares. This is because a limited company is legally separate from the owners/shareholders, so any debts the company runs up have nothing to do with the owner's personal assets. This is called limited liability and this is why they are called limited companies.

- All limited companies set up in the UK have a legal name that includes the word 'Limited' or 'Ltd' at the end.

Partnership

A partnership is much the same as a sole trader except that there is more than one owner. Each of the owners is called a partner.

- Just like a sole trader, the partners have unlimited liability for any debts that the partnership runs up.

- The partners have to agree how they will split any investments they make in the company, how much they will each get paid, how much time each of them will spend working in the business, and so on. They often do this by drawing up a partnership agreement between them.

- A partnership is more complex to set up than a sole trader because of the partnership agreement.

- Partners share the profits made by the partnership, as stated in the agreement, and then they pay tax on their share by completing self-assessment tax returns just like a sole trader.

Franchise

A franchise is a particular kind of business model where an established business or brand sells the rights to use their business name, logo, products and sales model. A small business that signs up to become a franchise can access some of the benefits of belonging to a large corporation but is still run and owned independently. For instance, one benefit might be advertising that a small business would never be able to afford. Examples of well-known franchise businesses are:

- McDonalds
- Costa Coffee
- Subway

Different franchises will have different rules about how each business has to operate and will have different start-up and on-going fees.

The previous three examples - sole trader, limited company and partnership - are legal structures that a business can take. A franchise is not a legal structure, which means that a sole trader, a partnership or a limited company can operate as a franchise business.

Chain

A chain is when a business opens mutliple branches with the same logos, branding and offering the same products or services. In a chain one business owns and directly operates all of the branches. This is the main difference bewteen a chain and franchise.

Like a franchise, a chain is not a legal structure - it is simply a type of business model.

Organisational policies

We have talked about some of the rules that an employer has to follow according the law. However there are many other rules, known as organisational policies, that a business may implement in order to run their business successfully. As long as these rules do not contradict any laws then businesses are free to decide upon them for themselves. Some typical policies are discussed below.

Health and safety

By law every business must have a health and safety policy in line with the Health and Safety at Work Act (1974). If there are five or more employees then this policy must be written down but in all cases it sets out the following:

- aims of the business relating to health and safety
- roles and responsibilities for health and safety within the business
- systems and procedures in place.

Complaints

At some point in its operation a business will have a customer who is dissatisfied with aspects of the business. Whilst not a legal requirement, a complaints policy will set out how a business will deal with these incidents.

A negative customer experience can have a negative impact on the business. For instance, they may never use the business again and may leave negative reviews, which might put other people off. However, dealing with a customer's complaints efficiently and sympathetically can even increase their trust in the business and their likelihood to recommend it to others. For these reasons it is useful to have a complaints policy.

A normal policy will state:

- how a customer can complain
- how the business will respond, including a timeframe for response
- how the problem might be solved - for instance, guaranteed money back if the the customer and business cannot agree on any other solution.

Dress code

Many companies have a dress code that sets out what is considered acceptable for members of staff. In some case this might be a specific uniform. In other cases it might be more general but state general standards that are acceptable and unacceptable - for instance 'smart shoes, no trainers'.

A dress code normally exists to ensure a certain level of professionalism is projected whilst at work and to make people feel part of a team. This is particularly important in any role where people are meeting members of the public or representing their company to third parties, but can still be important in non public-facing jobs.

115

A dress code must not, however, discriminate against anyone on the basis of their race, religion, gender, disability or anything else, in line with The Equality Act (2010).

Use of social media

Social media apps on smartphones allow people to send out information at any moment of the working day to hundreds or even thousands of people at the click of a button. This can be a problem for companies for the following reasons:

- Social media can be addictive to some people which means they can spend a lot of time checking or posting messages on their phone when they should be working.

- The employee represents the company they work for and their comments or posts might be mistaken as representing their company rather than their own opinions - particularly if these comments are made during the working day.

- Offensive material posted in personal accounts is likely to be completely unacceptable for most companies.

- It is easy to share confidential information, even by accident for instance in the background of a photograph. The company will wish some information to remain confidential for legal reasons or because they don't want to share it with competitors.

For these reasons, a company may have a social media policy which will cover things such as:

- how often employees check their accounts at work

- how posts, comments and replies could reflect badly on the company or put the company in a bad light

- ensuring no confidential information is ever revealed

- ensuring no offensive material is posted by an employee.

If an employee is expected to use social media on behalf of the business, for instance running a company account, then they will have additional responsibilites - such as not posting negative comments about competitors.

Attendance

Whilst an employee contract will cover the number of working hours and times, an attendance policy will go into greater detail. It will cover what rules are in place regarding situations such as:

- issues with punctuality, including arriving late and/or leaving early

- acceptable and unacceptable reasons for non-attendance

- procedures when an employee is sick - for instance how to communicate illness, how much notice is required

- procedures for excessive sick leave (e.g. number of days per year)

- procedures for extended periods of illness (e.g doctor's certificate required)

- compassionate leave policy (for instance, to attend a funeral)

Having all of these procedures and policies in place means that all employees know what is expected of them.

Store presentation

When working in retail the appearance of a shop projects an image to customers about the way the business is run. So retail businesses may also have a policy that states how the shop should look at all times. It normally concerns:

- how clean the shop is and how often it should be cleaned

- how tidy the shop is and how often it should be tidied

- how the shop should be arranged and how visible the various products should be - for instance, how regularly stock needs to be checked and re-stocked

- health and safety aspects, to reiterate how important they are and what to do (for instance, what to do in the event of a spillage, how to ensure no items could possibly fall and hurt someone).

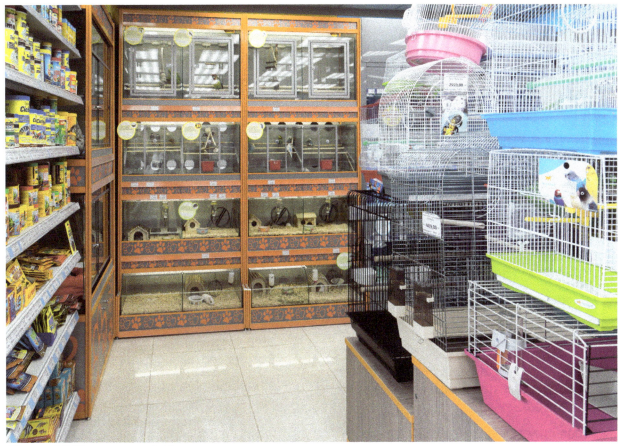

Figure 32 Store presentation

Professional standards

Whilst many of the previous policies cover specific issues, a professional standards policy is more general. It states what behaviour is expected from every employee of the company when representing them. This can include general behaviour such as:

- behaving respectfully towards all members of staff and the public

- displaying inclusive behaviour and using inclusive language

- being polite and moderate in tone and behaviour

- non-toleration of threatening, abusive or aggressive behaviour

It can also include:

- ensuring employees know, understand and follow all laws relevant to their work

- applying knowledge and training to the very best of an employee's abilities

- working hard and taking responsibility for actions

- working as part of a team

- to not be neglectful in any duties that are part of the role

For someone working in animal care a more specific professional standard might be to provide the best standards of care to all animals at all time.

Promotion of the organisation

Every business or organisation has to promote itself in some way. This might be because almost all businesses and organisations need people to interact with it in some way.

- It might be a business which needs to sell things in order to make profit, such as a pet shop.

- Or it might be a charity that needs people to make donations to help prevent animal cruelty.

There are lots of different ways to promote an organisation.

Displays

A display can be made of a number of different elements, including posters and leaflets. They often have one large eye-catching poster and perhaps some other visual elements such as photographs. There might also be a table containing further items of interest - as well as leaflets this might include further information sheets, books, and notepads as well as promotional items such as pens and badges to give away.

Displays at exhibitions would be manned by one or two people. Alternatively a smaller more permanent display in a local library might be left unattended.

Advantages

- good for attracting visitors - particularly if the display is manned

- a good place to give out or display other promotional material such as leaflets, website address etc.

- when targeted in the right place or at the right people, can lead to good new relationships with customers.

Disadvantages

- takes time to plan and set up

- can only run one or two displays at the same time - can only reach a very limited number of people

- all of the other promotional elements need to be created and set up as part of a display.

Posters

Posters are large enough that they can be seen from a distance. Well-designed posters catch people's attention in some way - often with striking images or with some large but simple phrases. They are normally used to convey one simple and clear piece of information.

Posters are displayed in areas where lots of people pass. Typical examples might be local libraries, cafes, schools or college, or within any organisation that has a similar audience. They are useful for advertising services, products or forthcoming events. You must

always ask permission before putting up any posters.

Advantages

- can be produced on a home computer

- easy to print off as many copies as are required

- good for conveying short, simple and easy-to-understand information.

Disadvantages

- needs access to a printer that uses larger sizes of paper

- printing lots of copies can get expensive, particularly if printing in full-colour

- information can go out of date

- time-consuming to find locations for posters and asking for permission

- limited number of people will see each poster, and only a few of them might actually act on it - and it is difficult to know how many of them did.

Leaflets

Leaflets are used when organisations want to include more information than in a poster. They often begin with a simple message or eye-catching image, and then follow up with a number of paragraphs of text.

Advantages

- cheaper to print than posters

- can be printed at home on A4 printers if necessary

- more space for information allows for greater detail

- can be sent through the post, put through people's letter boxes, left in cafes, shops and libraries (with permission).

Disadvantages

- may need to be printed professionally to give a better impression

- smaller, so their impact may be lost amongst other leaflets sharing the same space

- limited number of people will see each leaflet and difficult to know how many people have acted on a leaflet

- there is a cost of sending leaflets through the post.

Websites

A website is a great way to make information public. A website can be seen by anyone around the world who has access to the internet. It allows an organisation to place all their important information in one place, and then use their website address in all communications. Most people expect an organisation to have a website - if they don't then for some people the organisation is not real!

Advantages:

- a website can be updated immediately

- a website can be expanded as required - it can be a single page or hundreds of different pages, as required

- the potential audience is huge

- setting up a website is a relatively simple task

- websites allow you to track how many people visited each day.

Disadvantages:

- it can very difficult for new or small websites to feature in search engine results which can make it hard for people to find the website by accident

- this means that other forms of promotion may be needed to direct people to the website

- there is an annual fee for hosting a website (athough this is relatively small)

- whilst they are relatively simple to set up, writing and posting content requires someone who is comfortable with technology

- information must be kept up to date

- the website reflects the organisation, so it must look professional, but creating a professional-looking website will take

some time and may require some external expertise.

Social media

Social media refers to websites and apps such as Instagram, Facebook, Twitter and Snapchat. As well as being for personal use, businesses use them to promote themselves, to connect with potential customers or clients and for advertising.

Advantages:

- posting useful or relevant information will lead to new followers or connections that can help spread the word about the organisation

- there are groups on social media dedicated to most interests - so it is possible to find exactly the right people to target promotions to

- social media is free to use

- information is available about who interacted with what post or comment, so you can see how effective promotional messages are

- some posts can become very popular very quickly, reaching far more people than would be realistic using traditional promotional methods

- with most people using their smartphones for social media, followers can be reached and notified instantly - this is great for live updates or changes to plans.

Disadvantages:

- businesses have to be careful not to treat their social media channels as their personal social media accounts

- posts and comments can be seen by anyone on the platform - this means that all content must be very carefully considered before making public

- trends move very quickly - trying to predict or follow them can be difficult

- a great deal of time can be wasted checking accounts, replying to comments and posting messages, particularly if using more than one app

- there are people called trolls online who purposely pick arguments and post negative comments - dealing with such people can be upsetting and distract from the task itself

- business users can forget that getting 'likes' is not in itself the main objective!

- there is a cost to advertising on these platforms; and an advertising plan has to be carefully thought through before setting up any adverts.

Events

All sorts of events can be used for promotion. The subject of the event may not have anything to do with the organisation's work but instead provides an opportunity to meet people in person and introduce them to the organisation. An event is normally run by a number of people - the bigger the event the more people would be needed to run it.

Examples of self-organised events include:

- jumble sale

- fun run

- coffee morning

- raffle

- disco

- quiz night

- meet and greet - e.g. open the doors of a rescue shelter for the public to look around.

Alternatively you might simply attend an event organised by another organisation. Some examples of large events were given in Section 1.3 of this unit, but there are plenty of other smaller, local events that take place all around the country.

Advantages:

- great way to meet people interested in the organisation

- can have very detailed discussions with people about all aspect of the organisation

- opportunity to make personal connections and relationships.

Disadvantages:

- very time-consuming to set up one event

- a number of people will be needed to help prepare for the event and be present on the day

- even for a busy event there is limited time, and therefore only a limited number of people to talk to

- requires other promotional material to be effective.

Implications of social media

Use of personal social media

Using social media for promotion can lead to some confusion between personal and professional use. As previously discussed all comments, including personal ones, are a reflection of an employee's organisation and need to be carefully considered before posting. The use of social media for personal use at work may be covered by an organisational policy as previously discussed; but even if not then an employee should not spend time at work checking their personal social media accounts.

Negative social media comments

It is likely that an organisation will come across negative comments from time to time. Sometimes these comments may be justified, or be in the form of genuine complaints, in which case careful thought and attention must be given as how best to respond.

Other comments may be less genuine - in which case the best response is often to ignore them. There is no point in getting into a public argument with anyone about anything - it just reflects badly on the organisation.

All responses, as well as the original comments, are visible to everyone so it is important to be respectful, polite and calm at all times.

Your organisation may have particular policies in place to deal with these issues. You should make sure you are fully aware of any such policies or speak to your manager if in doubt.

120

e-safety

It is important that everyone keeps safe online. This includes using social media apps, interacting with all websites, using email and any interactions online using a computer or phone.

There are several dangers associated with online activity. They can be split into those that pose a risk to finances and personal informaton and those that pose a risk to personal safety.

Financial and personal information threats

With much activity now online, criminals have a number of ways to steal information and money from people, or simply disrupt people's lives.

- Malware - a general term for any software that is meant to disrupt or cause harm. Typical malware includes computer viruses, worms and Trojans. Malware is either spread through running infected programs, spread by connecting to infected networks or USB dives, or installed by accident when installing other software. The exact purpose of each depends but in all cases they can damage your computer or phone and pose a security threat.

- Social engineering is when criminals try to frighten or fool people into giving them confidential information or clicking on links which installs malware. This can be in the form of emails, text messages or phone calls pretending to be from a bank, or any organisation with which you have an account, They will often ask for your credit card details, or ask you to confrm your login details after clicking on a link. If you did, you would send your details directly to a criminal!

- In other cases these emails might simply ask for money - or pretend you have a fine which needs paying straight away.

- Criminals can also see communications when you are logged into public WiFi networks. You may not even realise they can see your confidential information being transmitted.

If criminals steal personal details from you then they can go on to steal money from you or even steal your identity. To prevent this from happening you should take note of the following guidelines.

- Do not open suspicious-looking emails, and attachments. Even if the sender's address looks familiar, if there's something strange about the message then do not open it.

- Never log in from a link in an odd-looking email. Always go direct to the website in a separate browser.

- A real bank or other organisation would never ask you for login information to be sent over an email or over the phone.

- Always ensure you have antivirus software installed (on your phone as well as you computer) and make sure it is completely up to date.

- Ensure your passwords are hard to guess and are changed on a regular basis.

Personal safety

Not everyone on the internet is who they say they are and not everyone's intentions are harmless. You should always be very careful about interacting with anyone who you do not know in real life.

Typical threats to personal safety are as follows.

- Cyberbullying - when people write offensive things, make threats, share embarrassing photographs or otherwise try to make someone feel ashamed or afraid.

- Trolling - when someone writes a comment trying to cause a reaction. They often do this by writing something rude, aggressive or offensive.

- People pretending to be someone else - they may do this to try and obtain personal information from you.

Steps you can take to stay safe include the following:

- Ensure you have looked at your privacy settings on all social media sites. You may be unwittingly allowing anyone on the site to see photographs, read information about you, find out your phone number and email address, and even where you live and work. Photographs may be tagged with your location, which can reveal a suprising amount about where you live and where you work.

- Be careful about what photographs you upload to social media. Even if you are sure only real-life friends can see them, remember that once uploaded these images pass from your possession into the company who owns the social media company. Friends may choose to forward photos to other people, and what might seem harmless now might cause problems or embarrassment in the future.

- Never reveal passwords or personal information to people over the internet. Remember that anyone you have never met in real life might be lying about their age, their gender and their interests.

- Don't reply to trolls or cyberbullies - block them instead. If you are upset or worried about cyberbullying then find a trusted adult to talk to.

- Never meet up with anyone in real life that you only know online. If anyone you don't know has asked you to meet up then tell a parent, your manager, a teacher or another adult.

- Some people use the internet and social media sites as a place to groom people for sexual abuse. If anyone is making you feel uncomfortable, acting strangely or pressuring you in any way then tell a parent, your manager, a teacher or another adult.

You can help ensure the safety of friends and others around you by acting kindly online, not forwarding photographs without permission and checking whether people want to be tagged in photographs before doing so.

Jargon Buster

assets anything of material value that belongs to someone

unlimited liability when there is no limit to how much debt that an individual could be responsible for

limited liability when there is a limit to how much debt that an individual could be responsible for

shareholders the owners of a limited company

trolls people on the internet who intentionally upset others

Quiz Questions

1 Describe the differences between a limited company and a sole trader.

2 Describe the advantages and disadvantages of using social media for promotion.

3 Define e-safety.

4 Describe some of the features that a company attendance policy might include.

Revision questions

1. Which of these is the most likely sign of shock?

a   Red mucuous membrane.
b   Discharge from the ears.
c   White mucous membrane.
d   Discharge from the nose.

2. Which of these parasites can only be found in fish?

a   Fleas
b   Ticks
c   Mites
d   Gill flukes

3. What routine care should be given to a hamster?

a   Teeth checked for plaque.
b   Teeth checked for gum disease.
c   Teeth checked for length.
d   Teeth checked for fillings.

4. Which of the following activities does **not** require a licence under the The Animal Welfare Regulations 2018?

a   Running a dog-grooming business.
b   Running a pet shop.
c   Running a dog day-care business.
d   Running a horse-riding school.

5. Which of these dogs are illegal to own under the Dangerous Dogs Act 1991?

a   Staffordshire Bull Terrier
b   Doberman
c   Rottweiler
d   Pit Bull Terrier

6. Which of these is **not** one of the five animal welfare needs?

a   Need for a suitable environment.
b   Need for appropriate stimulation.
c   Need to be able to exhibit normal behaviour patterns
d   Need for a suitable diet.

7. Which of the following is a bacterial disease?

a   Thrush
b   Avian flu
c   Kennel cough
d   Equine influenza

8. What is the most likely outcome if a puppy develops canine herpes virus?

a   They will die.
b   They will pass the virus on to their mother.
c   They will pass the virus on to humans.
d   They will develop symptoms such as coughing and sneezing.

9. What is the best way of preventing leptospirosis?

a   Vaccination.
b   Separating animals so they don't spread it bewteen them.
c   Preventing animals from foraging for food.
d   Keeping food sources free from mice and rats.

10. A dog suffers repeated fits. Which disorder are they likely to have?

a   Cushing's syndrome.
b   Stress.
c   Pica.
d   Epilepsy.

11. Which of these is **not** one of the three aims of first aid?

a   Preserve life.
b   Prevent ill-health.
c   Prevent situation from deteriorating.
d   Prevent suffering.

12. What legislation covers the activities that are allowed under first aid?

a   Veterinary Surgeons Act 1966.
b   The First Aid Act 1998
c   The Animal Welfare Act 2006
d   The Animal Welfare Regulations 2018.

13. What condition is caused by an animal's body becoming too hot?

a   Convulsion
b   Hypothermia
c   Colic
d   Hyperthermia

14. After introducing a new houseplant, the family cat has been vomiting and displaying signs of stomach pain. What should you do?

a   Give the cat some extra food.
b   Try and make the cat vomit again before ringing the vet.
c   Wait and see if the cat gets better.
d   Make the cat comfortable, note the species of houseplant and call the vet immediately.

15. A dog has been involved in a fight. It has sustained some scratches and bite marks but they don't require further treatment. Immediately afterwards you notice the dog coughing up blood. What is this most likely to indicate?

a   That the dog is bleeding internally
b   That the dog has lost some teeth.
c   That the dog swallowed the other dog's blood.
d   That the dog has some other health condition.

16. Which of these is **not** a preserved food?

a   Grass.
b   Hay.
c   Pellets
d   Silage.

17 Which nutrient plays an important part in repairing animal muscles and tissues?

a   Fat.
b   Carbohydrate.
c   Vitamin C.
d   Protein.

18. A cat food label in a rescue centre states that it is 'suitable for feeding after parturition'. Which animal should it be fed to?

a   A kitten.
b   An older cat.
c   A new mother.
d   An injured cat.

19. Why might a farmer decide to install automatic feeders on her farm?

a   Because it will reduce the amount of food consumed.
b   The farm workers will no longer need to fill the feeders, leaving them to get on with other jobs.
c   Because they cost less than manual feeders.
d   Because they can be filled up wth more food less frequently than manual feeders, giving the farm workers more time to do other things.

20 Which of the following has the highest nutritional energy requirements?

a   A recently retired labrador police dog.
b   A healthy adult male labrador.
c   A lactating female labrador.
d   A preganant female labrador.

21. What nutritional benefit does grit provide to a budgerigar?

a   Provides vitamin A for digestion.
b   Has no nutritional benefit.
c   Helps to maintain feathers.
d   Provides calcium for strong bones.

22. Which of the following is the most suitable way to store animal food?

a   In sealed containers left by the window.
b   In sealed containers in a locked, dry room.
c   In sealed containers in a damp room.
d   In open containers in a dry cellar.

23. You notice a goldfish swimming on one side. What would be an appropriate course of action?

a   Immediately move the fish into its own tank.
b   Change the water of the current tank.
c   Wait for a few days to see if it gets better.
d   Consult the feeding records to check if there have been any changes of diet.

24. A dog that eats stones has what condition?

a   Pica.
b   Coprophagia.
c   Malnutrition.
d   Obesity.

25. Which of these would you associate with animal accommodation made from wood?

a   Safe to leave in the rain untreated.
b   Easy to clean.
c   Resistant to gnawing.
d   Easy to work into different shapes.

26. Which is the most important aspect to consider when housing a crested gecko in a vivarium?

a   The vivarium should look attractive.
b   The temperature and humidity should be carefully monitored.
c   The gecko should be visible at all times.
d   There should be a good range of plastic toys available.

27. What is the most suitable layout for a rabbit hutch?

a   One single uncovered living area placed outdoors.
b   One single covered living area placed outdoors
c   One single uncovered living area placed indoors
d   A covered living area made up of a number of different areas and hides.

28. Which of these is the **least** important consideration for day accommodation at a verterinary surgery?

a   There is plenty of space to exercise.
b   The accommodation is clean and hygienic.
c   It provides a stress-free environment.
d   It is fully secure.

29. Which of these properties of a substrate is **most** suitable for a pet rat kept in a centrally-heated house?

a   Odour-controlling properties.
b   Insulating properties.
c   Non-slip properties.
d   Bio-degradable properties.

30. Which of the following is the correct way to fully clean a surface?

a   Apply disinfectant and rinse.
b   Apply disinfectant, clean and rinse, apply detergent and leave before rinsing.
c   Apply disinfectant, clean and rinse, apply detergent and immediately rinse.
d   Apply detergent, clean and rinse, apply disinfectant and leave before rinsing.

31. If you have an accident at work which legislation should you refer to?

a   COSHH.
b   RIDDOR.
c   PPE.
d   Health and Safety at Work Act (1974).

32. A syringe that has been used to inject a cow is classified as which of the following?

a   Non-hazardous waste.
b   Biodegradable waste
c   Hazardous waste.
d   Recyclable waste.

33. What is the correct term for an animal that is most active at dawn and dusk?

a   Nocturnal.
b   Diurnal.
c   Biurnal.
d   Crepuscular.

34. Which of the following is the best way to approach a strange dog?

a   Walk head-on directly towards the dog.
b   Stand still and stare at the dog until it looks away.
c   Approach calmly and slowly from the side .
d   Talk loudly whilst walking towards the dog.

35. What might cause atypical behaviour in a solitary animal species?

a   A lack of sunlight.
b   Being forced to live with other animals.
c   Looking after offspring.
d   Searching for food.

36. Communciation between two animals of the same species is known as what?

a   Infraspecfic communicaton.
b   Intraspecific communication.
c   Interspecific communication.
d   Interrelated communication.

37. Stereotypy is an example of what?

a   A medical disorder.
b   A stress-related disorder.
c   Typical behaviour.
d   Auditory communication.

38. Which species demonstrate the highest levels of parental care?

a   Horses.
b   Zebra fish.
c   Tortoise.
d   Corn snake.

39. Which of the following might explain differences in territorial behaviour between male and female deer?

a   Mating males and females stay together for life.
b   There is only one dominant adult female in the deer social stucture.
c   There is only one dominant adult male in the deer social stucture.
d   There are no young in the deer social structure.

40. The male and female looking after their young is called:

a   Intensive parental care.
b   Maternal care.
c   Parental care.
d   Biparental care

41. For which of the following would video camera observations be most appropriate?

a   Sociable animals.
b   Solitary animals.
c   Shy animals.
d   Large animals.

42. An observation of tigers in a zoo takes place every morning for 20 minutes. This is an example of what?

a   An ethogram.
b   Instantaneous scan sampling.
c   Ad lib sampling.
d   Focal sampling.

43. Which item of equipment would be most suitable for an aggressive feral cat that required injections?

a   A noose.
b   A muzzle.
c   A crush cage.
d   A towel.

44. Why is enrichment important?

a   To ensure an animal is eating the correct nutrients.
b   To prevent obesity.
c   To provide stimulation.
d   To socialise animals.

45. A 17 year old works in a pet shop for 6 hours. What is the minimum rest break they are entitled to each day?

a   20 minutes.
b   30 minutes
c   40 minutes.
d   60 minutes

46. A trainee catttery worker would **not** be expected to perform which of the following tasks?
a   Clean out the cages.
b   Answer the phone.
c   Supervise another member of staff.
d   Feed the animals.

47. What is the PDSA's main aim?

a   To rescue stray animals.
b   To represent the health and welfare interests of dogs.
c   To prevent cruelty to animals.
d   To provide low-cost health care to animals.

48. Who is the BSAVA Congress aimed at?

a   Veterinary professionals specialising in farm animals.
b   Veterinary professionals specialising in zoo animals.
c   Veterinary surgeons.
d   Veterinary professionals specialising in companion animals.

49. A member of the public spills a hot drink whilst visiting an animal rescue centre. Who is responsible for reporting the incident?

a   The most senior member of staff.
b   Any member of staff who sees the spillage.
c   The member of the public who spilt it.
d   The owner of the rescue centre.

50. A company that uses national or international branding, but is not owned by the brand, is known as a what?

a   A franchise.
b   A limited company.
c   A chain.
d   A sole trader.

51. Why might a company have a complaints procedure?

a   It is a legal requirement.
b   To ensure a complaint is resolved smoothly.
c   So it can be sent to any customer who complains.
d   So the compaint can be passed on to someone else.

52. A zoo needs to make sure that all visitors and staff sanitise their hands properly before entering and after leaving the premises. What would be the best way to communicate this?

a   On social media.
b   Through the zoo's website.
c   By printing some leaflets.
d   By displayng posters at the entrance and exit.

53. Someone posts a negative comment about the rescue centre in which you work on a social media account. What should you do?

a   Reply immediately using the centre's account, telling them they are wrong.
b   Wait until the next day, then reply using the centre's account, asking them to never visit again.
c   Do nothing and discuss the post with your manager.
d   Reply using your personal account.

54. Which of the following is **not** an e-safety risk?

a   Posting your address on a social media account.
b   Liking a friend's post.
c   Clicking on a link in an email from a stranger.
d   Not checking your privacy settings on a social media account.

Scenario

Whilst walking home from work you wtiness a German Shepherd, which has been let off the lead, attacking and injuring a Jack Russell. The Jack Russell and German Shepherd have sustained injuries. You have your first aid box with you.

55. The owner of the German Shepherd is in breach of which part of the Dangerous Dogs Act 1991?

a   He let the dog off the lead in a public place.
b   The dog should have been muzzled.
c   The dog was out of control and causing a danger.
d   The dog was on the list of banned breeds.

56. The Jack Rusell has a bite wound to the neck and is losing blood. What should you do first?

a   Begin wrapping a bandage around the wound whilst asking someone to ring the police to report the owner.
b   Ring a veterinary surgery, clean the wound and then apply a dressing.
c   Ask someone to ring a veterinary surgery, check that the German Shepherd has been restrained, and then carefully approach the Jack Rusell with the aim of stopping the bleeding.
d   Tell the owner what first aid they should apply and ring the veterinary surgery to report the incident

57. As well as bleeding, the Jack Rusell is likely to show signs of what condition?

a   Shock.
b   Hypothermia.
c   Colic.
d   Hyperthermia.

58. The German Shepherd is still showing signs of aggression. What body language would you expect to see?

a   Ears flat, mouth half open, tail down.
b   Ears forward, lips curled, tail up.
c   Ears forward, mouth closed, tail up.
d   Ears up, mouth open, head on one side.

59. You find out later that a charitable organisation has rehomed the German Shepherd. Which organisation is most likely to have been involved?

a   The Kennel Club.
b   BNVA.
c   Defra.
d   RSPCA

.

NOTE: These questions are designed for practice only. They may differ from any actual assessments.

Index

Lightning Source UK Ltd.
Milton Keynes UK
UKHW051012050522
402505UK00004B/50

9 780992 900243